Manual of

for

Undergraduates

MW00980955

Manual of Anaesthesia for Undergraduates

DR. SATISH G. DESHPANDE
Professor & Head
Department of Anaesthesiology
S.R.T.R. Medical College
Ambajogai, Distt. Beed, Maharashtra

CBS

CBS PUBLISHERS & DISTRIBUTORS
NEW DELHI • BANGALORE

ISBN : 81-239-1493-8

First Edition : 2007

Published by :
Satish Kumar Jain for CBS Publishers & Distributors,
4596/1-A, 11 Darya Ganj, New Delhi - 110 002 (India)
E-mail : cbspubs@vsnl.com • Website : www.cbspd.com

Branch Office :
2975, 17th Cross, K.R. Road,
Bansankari 2nd Stage, Bangalore - 560070
Fax : 080-26771680 • E-mail : cbsbng@vsnl.net

Publishing Director : Vinod K. Jain

Printed at :
India Binding House, Noida (UP).

Preface

Amongst the medical fraternity subjects, Anaesthesiology remains ignored branch and the personalities are denoted as characters working behind the curtain. Anaesthesiology is deprived off its presence from the MBBS curriculum. Previously it was considered as a part of surgery branch but since 1846 due to inspection of first successful public demonstration, it started to be included as the branch of medical fraternity.

Now Anaesthesiology has gained tremendous importance and the persons working in the specialty have proved their presence as team leader in all emergency services. Although working behind the curtain as in closed operation theater, now many branches concerned to subject have opened their doors for anaesthesiologists as Pain Clinic, Intensive Care Unit, Intensive Respiratory Care Unit, Disaster Management, etc. where working has proved its significance.

No doubt after obtaining MBBS degree, those obtaining postgraduate qualification in Anaesthesiology have shown their expertise, clinically with adequate academic literature. To be expert in the subject, there is adequate clinical and academic literature for postgraduate students and practicing anaesthesiologists.

As like the parent subject, the available literature is also somewhat ignored and till now only postgraduate curriculum was considered. Again one more problem concerned to the subject is that, it is not considered as the subject to be taught and studied at undergraduate level, hence there is no clinical exposure for students, there is no importance of subject even at the MBBS examination (Practical and Theory) so the literature of the subject covering undergraduate curriculum is also lagging behind.

Now some medical universities of India are reviving and

considering the subject to have its significance and importance so starting to add some questions in theory or even to have separate theory section for examination. Now some questions related to clinical anaesthesia, resuscitation and critical care are being included in the Postgraduate CET examination.

At undergraduate level the students search the literature or some topics from the reference books specifically meant for postgraduate students and were unable to get knowledge from the vast postgraduate literature. It is beyond their capacity to get required knowledge from the books and wasting their time in the search in the books which are mainly for the postgraduate studies.

Hence I am sure this book will definitely find way between the requirement of medical undergraduates to fulfill their academic achievements. It is sincere effort from my side to provide a comprehensive but adequate knowledge palatable for undergraduate students, the topics of importance at the time of examination, even at clinical practice as well as the topics of importance at every aspect of medical practice. As there is no such type of book available for undergraduate students to fulfill academic and clinical demands of undergraduate students. In short this book is covering History part of Anaesthesia, Induction anaesthetic agents, Inhalational agents, Neuromuscular blocking agents, Preanaesthesia preparation and medication, Anaesthesia machine, Endotracheal intubation technique, Spinal and epidural anaesthesia, Monitoring during anaesthesia, Intraoperative and postoperative complications, Cardio-respiratory resuscitation, Day care anaesthesia, Role of anaesthesiologist outside operation theater, etc.

At undergraduate level there is less requirement of deep knowledge about anaesthesia but everyone should know at least the basic concepts but the undergraduate student should feel that I have touched the subject and so that it will be easier for them to think of taking the subject for their postgraduate curriculum. So it will be definite guide for the undergraduates to have basic and comprehensive knowledge about the subject.

Dr. Satish Deshpande (M. D.)
Professor and Head
Department of Anaesthesiology
SRTR Medical College
Ambajogai, Distt. Beed (MS)

Contents

1

History of Anaesthesia

The developments in Anaesthesiology branch since its introduction in 1846 has been erratic, long period of stagnation being occasionally broken by improvements and advances. Anaesthesia as we know today was first time used by W.T.G. Morton of Boston, who gave Ether at the Massachusets General Hospital on 16th October 1846 to Gilbert Abbott.

The technical difficulties associated with the administration of Ether were partly curtailed down by the substitution with Choloroform by J.V. Simpson Prof. of Obstetrics and Gynecology. John Snow was the first person to attempt with new anaesthetic agents and methods of their administration via apparatus. In 1863, Nitrous oxide was introduced in anaesthesia practice by G.O. Colton. During the next 40 to 50 years, there were few significant changes in the practice of anaesthesia but after 1920 the progress in the field quickened. In 1920, Ether and Chloroform were the main agents used but Ethyl chloride and Nitrous oxide were often employed for induction for which Simpson's open drop method was popular.

In 1917, first Boyle's anaesthesia machine appeared in the practice. Endotracheal technique by I.W. Magill and E. Stanley Rowbotham was introduced. Controlled respiration was introduced by H. Griffith in 1942. Local anaesthesia made its appearance in 1884 by Carl Koller. Spinal anaesthesia was first described by August Bier in 1898 and extradural block by F. Cathelin in 1901.

Technical improvements were slowly accompanied by academic recognition. The first examination of diploma was conducted in London in 1935 and in 1937 R.R. MacIntosh became first Professor of Anaesthesia.

Enormous developments in the use of monitoring equipments, high sophistication has taken place since last 20 years in the field of Anaesthesiology.

Milestones in Anaesthesia

1516 : Curare – South African arrow poison described by Petter Martyr Angherious

1540 : Valerius Cordus synthesized sweet oil of vitriol (Ether)

1628 : W.M. Harvey described circulation of blood.

1662 : Robert Boyle described Gas law relationship of volume and pressure of the gas.

1751 : Anaesthesia defined as a defect of sensation

1754 : Carbon dioxide was discovered by Von Helmont and was isolated by Black.

1771 : Discovery of Oxygen by Pristley and Carl Wilhelm Scheele independently

1777 : A. Lavoisier named the new air of Pristley as Oxygen.

1787 : J. Charles showed relationship of volume to the temperature of gas.

1800 : Davy described analgesic properties of Nitrous oxide and named it as laughing gas

1806 : Wilhelm Adam Serturner isolated morphine from opium

1816 : Rene Laennac invented stethoscope

1831 : Chloroform discovered independently by Von Liebeg and Guthrie
Atropine was prepared by Mein, Geiger and Hesse.

1842 : W.E. Clark gave ether for dental extraction.

1844 : Horace Wells introduced nitrous oxide inhalation to produce anaesthesia during dental extraction.

1846 : W.T.G. Mortan demonstrated anaesthetic properties of ether on 16th October

The word anaesthesia was suggested by Oliver Wendell Holmes for Mortan's etherisation.

19th Dec. tooth extracted by Dr.Boott,, ether was given by Mr. Robinson

21st Dec. first surgical operation in England under ether anaesthesia by Robert Listen.

1847 : James Simpson introduced chloroform in clinical practice for pain relief in labour.

John Snow published first book on the inhalation of ether in surgical operation.

1849 : First anaesthesia death due to chloroform, 10th oct. St. Thomas Hospital.

1853 : Pravaz invented glass syringe. Hypodermic syringe and needle invented by Alexander Wood

1857 : Claude Bernard showed that curare acts on myoneural junction

1860 : Albort Nieman purified alkaloid and given the name cocaine

1868 : Edmund Andrews combined oxygen with nitrous oxide

1880 : Wiliam Macewan, surgeon introduced tracheal intubation by mouth.

1881 : Fredrick Trendlenburg, Prof of surgery introduced head down tilt with pelvic elevation for abdominal surgery.

1882 : Synthesis of Cyclopropane by Von Fruend

1884 : Koller demonstrated local anaesthetic properties of cocaine on cornea

Wm. Stewart Halsted and Hall gave first nerve block with cocaine,Mandibular nerve.

1885 : J.L. Corning neurologist produced analgesia by accidental subarachnoid injection of cocaine.

1888 : First Hydrabad Chloroform commission

1889 : Second Hydrabad Chloroform commission—reports stated that chloroform is not cardiac depressant.

1890 : Redard introduced Ethyl chloride for local analgesia

1895 : W.K. Roentgen discovered X-rays.

1898 : August Bier introduced first successful clinical spinal analgesia.

1900 : Karl Landsteiner described ABO blood grouping.

1904 : Procaine was synthesized by Alford Einhorn

1905 : First society of anaesthesist formed in USA

1910 : Elmer Ira Mackesson introduced first on-demand intermittent flow gas and oxygen machine. Arthur Lawen described extradural analgesia.

1911 : A.E. Guedel reported technique of self administration of nitrous oxide in obstetrics.

1912 : A. Lawen used curare to produce relaxation

1917 : Edmund Boyle described portable nitrous oxide / oxygen apparatus, chloroform bottle added in 1920.

1920 : Magill and RowBotham developed Endotracheal anaesthesia.

1923 : Carbon dioxide absorption technique was used by Waters'

1926 : J.S. Lundy put concept of balanced anaesthesia.

1928 : I.A. Magill introduced blind nasal intubation.

1930 : Brian Sword introduced circle method of carbon dioxide absorption.

1931 : A.M.D. Dogliotti re-introduced extradural analgesia.

1934 : J.S. Lundy introduced Thiopentone.
Ralph Waters reported use of Cyclopropane.

1937 : R.R. MacIntosh appointed as first Professor of Anaesthesia.

1940 : Development of controlled breathing by Guedel and NoseWorthy.

1942 : Griffith used curare in anaesthesia.

1943 : MacIntosh described curved laryngoscope blade

1947 : First clinical use of Lignocaine by Gordth

1956 : First examination in anaesthesia faculty

1966 : Ketamine used clinically by De Castro

1917 : Original Boyles' machine was introduced

1920 : Addition of vaporizing bottle to flow meters

1926 :   Addition of second vaporizing bottle and bypass control

1927 :   Addition of third water-tight feed tube for carbon dioxide

1930 :   Addition of plunger device

1933 :   Dry bobbin type of flow meter displaced water tight feed

1937 :   Rotameters displaced by dry bobbin flow meter

1878 :   Wm. MacEwen passed a tube from the mouth into the trachea using his fingers as a guide in conscious patient.

1850 :   Claude Bernard showed that curare acts by paralyzing the myoneural junction.

1935 :   King isolated d-tubocurarine from the crude drug and established chemical structure.

1942 :   H.R. Griffith gave curare for muscle relaxation.

1947 :   Bovet described Gallamine triethiodide

1949 :   Daniel Bovet introduced Suxamethonium.

1880 :   Rothenstein introduced Ethyl chloride spray.

1943 :   Lofgren and Lundqviest synthesized Lignocaine

1901 :   Nerve blocks were described by Harvey cushing

1885 :   J.L. Corning neurologist gave first spinal anaesthesia.

1898 :   16th August Bier gave first planned spinal block for surgery.

1901 :   M. Cathelin deliberately produced epidural block by caudal route

1895 :   Cushing and Codman introduced ether cards.

1910 :   MedKesson developed first practical intermittent flow, nitrous oxide/oxygen

anaesthesia machine.

1928 :   Foregger constructed first modern carbon dioxide absorption canister

1926 :   Brian and Sword invented circle filter system.

1913 :   Hewitt introduced pharyngeal airway.

1595 :   Sir Walter Raleigh reported use of arrow poison by Orinoco Indian tribes

1815 :   Watterton and Brodie showed curare can kill by asphyxia.

1935 :   King isolated d-tubocurarine from extracts

1930 : Introduction of circle system of Co_2 absorption by Brian Sword

1947 : L. Hewer and C.F. Hedfield introduced Trichloroethylene

1951 : C.W. Suckling synthesized Halothane.

1956 : M. Johnstone used Halothane clinically.

1904 : T.D. Buchana developed first department of anaesthesia and then became professor

1967 : Pancuronium was introduced.

1980 : Vecuronium and Atracurium were introduced in anaesthesia practice.

1990 : Pipecuronium and Doxacurium were introduced.

1996 : An atracuronium isomer Cistracurium was introduced. Rapacurium under trial.

Historical developments

- The first : 1846-1850 – Ether on folded towel
- Era of cone inhalers : 1850-1876
- Era of closed inhalers : 1876-19 06
- Era of open method of administration : 1895-1945
- Regression to semi-open method : 1905-1941
- Vapor method : 1867-1941
- Endotracheal anaesthesia : 1871-1945
- Gas anaesthesia : 1894-1945

The discovery of surgical anaesthesia is an American contribution and called as greatest contribution in medicine. Horace Wells a dentist of Hartford attended a sideshow in which Colton the chemist demonstrated the effects of nitrous oxide. There was no pain experienced by injured person. Wells was so impressed by the insensibility produced by the gas and decided to use in dental extraction. Wells continued to use the agent in his practice and became well known for his painless dentistry. Then he invited for demonstration in major operation in Massachusetts General Hospital, Boston. In his experiment, Wells failed to realize the pharmacological nature of nitrous oxide and demonstration was failure. He then became ether addict. Later he committed suicide in New York by cutting his cubital vein with hand in warm water bath.

First use – long

Crawford W Long first witnessed the effects of ether at frolics in Philadelphia. In January 1942, he administered the vapors of ether to James Venable. The method was successful and a large tumor was removed from the neck. The country people ignored the work.

First Demonstration

W.T.G. Morton born in Charleston, had consuming ambition to be a physician. He was forced to practice dentistry and came across with Wells. He consulted with Prof. Charles Jackson and learned that sulphuric ether had some effect in producing unconsciousness.

As a second year medical student, he obtained permission from John Collins Warren, the Prof. of surgery to make a public trial of ether for a major operation. The demonstration was set on 16th October 1846. It was turning point in history of anaesthesia. The name of patient was Gilbert Abbott. The operation was done by Dr. Warren, it was quiet, no struggle or screaming. Morton was named as discoverer of Surgical anaesthesia. Morton went through many trials and hardships there after. The public maligned him.

Dr. Oliver Holmes suggested the term "anaesthesia". This signifies insensibility for touch.

After civil war, Morton returned to Massachusetts. One day he received copy of an article written by Jackson in monthly magazine. It was full of hatred and claimed that Morton had nothing to do with the discovery of ether. He was enraged and suffered a mild stroke and went to New York and on July 15th it was afurnece, the Riverside hotel where Morton was staying. So he drive through central park in the evening to steady his nerves. Part way through, he grew giddy and weak, then just before carriage reached the park gates he reigned up the horses, jumped to the ground and soon fell unconscious in his wife's arms beneath a tree. He was taken to hospital and there died of his apoplexy.

Approximately after 100 years modern anaesthesia began around 1940. The first change in direction was the initial use of curare product of Griffith in 1942. The major inhaled anaesthetic substitutes included the non-inflammable, highly lipid soluble and potent vapors of halogenated inhalants, more versatile neuromuscular blocking agents were introduced.

2

Medical Gases Used in Anaesthesia

AIR

- Atmospheric air contains 78.08% Nitrogen, 20.95% Oxygen, 0.03% Carbon dioxide, 0.93% Argon with traces of neon, helium, krypton, hydrogen and xenon.
- Medical air is supplied in gray cylinders with black and white shoulder quadrants, compressed to 137 bar.
- It may be supplied through pipeline at 4 bar pressure.
- It is used as a respired gas and to drive ventilators.
- It also drives surgical drills.
- It has less impurities than industrial compressed air. It is not sterile.

OXYGEN

Oxygen is one of the basic essentials for maintenance of life. In 1771, J. Pristley discovered oxygen and named as dephlogisticated air. Lavoisier gave the name "Oxygen". Beddoes introduced oxygen therapy in 1794.

- It is manufactured by fractional distillation of liquid air.
- Boiling point is 183ºC.
- Molecular weight is 32
- Solubility in water – 0.024/ml at 37ºC

9

- Critical pressure – 52.8 bar
- Specific gravity – 1105
- It may ignite in presence of grease or oil.

Oxygen cylinders have black body with white shoulder and pressure is 1980 psi.Compressed oxygen in gas is more dangerous than in liquid form so on large scale requirement liquid oxygen is prepared. One liter of liquid oxygen yields 850 ml of gas oxygen. It is supplied in pipeline at pressure of 60 psi.

Clinical uses of oxygen

- Coronary vasodilatation in acute myocardial infarction
- To relieve peripheral vessel spasm
- Acute pulmonary disease – pneumonitis
- Cardiac decompensation
- Chronic pulmonary disease – bronchial asthma, chronic bronchitis
- Pulmonary oedema
- High altitude flying
- Postoperative excitement and delirium
- Postoperative distention of abdomen
- Migraine

Factors contributing for hypoxia

- General patients' factors
- Low atmospheric breathing mixture
- Ventilatory insufficiency
- Efficiency of oxygen intake is less
- Transport propel – haemoglobin and blood volume
- Degree of shunting
- Tissue uptake – oxygen consumption and arterio-venous oxygen difference

Hypoxia may be produced during or postoperatively in anaesthesia practice. There are variety of factors responsible for hypoxia in the patients. Before presenting the patients with clinical features of oxygen lack, oxygen supplementation should be under taken. It may be for treatment, preventive or anticipated purpose.

Oxygen therapy is under taken to restore tissue oxygen tension towards normal. It is most important life saving measure in cases with low blood oxygen tension, shock, severe haemorhage, coronary thrombosis, pulmonary oedema, heart failure, head injury, chest injury, etc. It is also used to dilute other anaesthetic gases and inhalational agents.

Methods of oxygen therapy

It may be administered by nasal catheter, poly mask, venti mask, oxygen tents, ventilators or Boyles' machine. Nasal catheter provides oxygen flow of 3 lit/min to raise inspired oxygen 30–60% and alveolar oxygen concentration up to 14–27%. Oxygen tents are beneficial in paediatric patients. Oxygen therapy devices may be fixed performance or variable performance devices.

Oxygen therapy without indication is also harmful and there may be dangerous oxygen toxicity. When administered in therapeutic range, oxygen does not have any untoward effects but 100% when administered for prolonged time, without any early beneficial effects it may produce irritation of respiratory tract. There may be chest pain, sore throat, congestion of eyes and nose, tingling and numbness, dizziness, nausea and vomiting. When administered in high-inspired concentration, it may cause myocardial depression, vaso-constriction, Co_2 narcosis, convulsions and pulmonary oedema and retrolental fibroplasias.

Hyperbaric oxygen therapy is indicated in carbon monoxide poisoning, cerebral oedema, gas gangrene, myocardial infarction, neonatal asphyxia, and chronic osteomylitis. The toxic effects of oxygen therapy are more common after hyper baric oxygen therapy.

CARBON DIOXIDE

Carbon dioxide was discovered by Von Helmant and isolated by J. Black in 1757. Usually it is produced by respiration, combustion and fermentation.

- It is colourless gas with pungent odour in high concentration.
- Molecular weight is 44
- Boiling point is 78.5°C
- Solubility in water is 0–88 ml/ml at 20°C
- Critical temperature is 31°C
- Critical pressure is 73.8 bar
- Specific gravity is 1520 and density is 1.87 kg/cc at 15°C

It is obtained from four sources :

- From fermentation in brewing of beer
- By product of manufacture of hydrogen in petroleum refining
- From combustion of fuels
- By heating magnesium and calcium carbonate in presence of their oxides It is stored in Gray cylinders at 50 bar pressure. Solid Co_2 is stored and transported in isolated containers.

Oxygen : Carbon dioxide premixed cylinders are available in various combinations.

Inspired air contains 0.03%, mixed expired gas 3.5–4% and alveolar gas 5.6% of CO_2. It is non-inflammable and does not support combustion.

Carbon dioxide stimulates respiration both in rate and depth due to direct stimulation of respiratory center and by reflex action on carotid and aortic bodies. An increase in partial pressure of 3 mm in blood, increases the tidal exchange by 100% and a decrease of 4 mm of Hg may cause apnoea.

Higher concentrations above 10%, it may cause dyspnoea, distress and headache, it produces narcosis at 30% concentration and at 40% causes stoppage of respiration.

The systemic blood pressure, cardiac output and heart rate progressively increases with rise in $PaCo_2$ At high $PaCo_2$, there is cardiovascular depression, cutaneous, coronary, cerebral vasodilatation with hypercpania and vasoconstriction with hypocapnia.

Clinical uses

- To increase depth of anaesthesia with volatile anaesthetic agents by stimulating respiration centrally.
- To produce hyperventilation, there by wider opening of glottis and ease of blind nasal intubation.
- To increase cerebral blood flow during carotid artery surgery.
- To stimulate onset of respiration
- In production of hyperaemia by vasodilatation
- To avoid hypocarbia in cardiopulmonary bypass
- To distend abdomen during laproscopy
- Cryosurgery
- In production laser light for surgical procedures.

Disadvantages and complications

- It is potent stimulant of sympathetic nervous system
- It increases cerebral blood flow and intra-cranial pressure
- It sensitizes myocardium to exogenous adrenaline.
- It reduces alveolar oxygen concentration
- In high concentration it produces narcosis.
- Now a days use of Carbon dioxide is obscured and it has no place in recent practice of anaesthesia.

NITROUS OXIDE

Pristley firstly prepared nitrous oxide in 1772. Anaesthetic properties were suggested by Sir Humphry Davy in 1779. Colton and Horace Wells first used it for painless tooth extraction in 1844.

- It is colourless inert gas and 1.5 times heavier than air
- It is sweat smelling, non-irritating to respiratory tract
- Molecular weight is 44
- It is stored as compressed liquid at 750 psi. The colour of cylinder is blue.
- It is non-inflammable, non-explosive but support combustion.
- Boiling point is 88°C

- Blood/gas solubility coefficient is 0–47 and oil/water coefficient is 3.2
- It may contain Nitric oxide and Nitrogen dioxide as impurities.
- Commercially it is manufactured by heating ammonium nitrate to 240°C then collected, purified and compressed in blue cylinders at 651 atmosphere
- It is filled 4/5 or ¾ of cylinder capacity. The cylinders are usually kept upright.
- During use, the cylinder cools due to latent heat of vaporization of the liquid and ice may form at lower part of the cylinder.
- Reducing valve is necessary to control the release of gas from cylinder.
- Nitrous oxide is less soluble in blood so the induction and recovery from anaesthesia is slow.
- Nitrous oxide reduces the MAC of other volatile anaesthetic agents by 50% and results in speedy induction. When administered along with Halothane, it increases the alveolar concentration of Halothane. This is called as second gas effect.

Pharmacological actions

- It causes depression of central nervous system due to oxygen displacement from cerebral cells.
- It has no direct effect on cardiovascular system and heart. Rarely it has negative inotropic and chronotropic effects on heart. It produces α-adrenergic stimulation of peripheral circulation. Slightly it increases peripheral vascular resistance and pulmonary vascular resistance.
- There is no direct effect on respiratory and muscular systems.
- There is no effect on liver and kidney functions.
- It is very stable and not affected by soda lime.
- It is eliminated via lungs within 2 minutes after stoppage.
- It is potent analgesic and weak anaesthetic gas.

Clinical uses

- It is used as sole anaesthetic agent for short surgical procedures along with oxygen.
- It is mainly used as a carrier gas with volatile anaesthetic agents
- As an analgesic in mixture of gases
- Obstetric analgesia
- Dental anaesthesia

Adverse effects and contraindications

It is non-toxic but on prolonged administration there may be bone marrow depression and agranulocytosis.

Prolonged nitrous oxide anaesthesia may cause diffusion of gas into the body cavities like brain, pleural cavity, middle ear, nasal sinuses, etc. This increases the volume and pressure of air and causes harmful effects. It diffuses more rapidly than nitrogen and distend gas filled cavities as 30 times more soluble than nitrogen.

It may produce distension of stomach if inhaled for prolonged time which is contributing factor in postoperative nausea and vomiting.

Following nitrous oxide anaesthesia, high percentage of expired volume may consists of nitrous oxide, so outward diffusion of gas lowers alveolar partial pressure of oxygen and thus diffusion hypoxia may develop or Fink effect in early postoperative period. It is prevented by oxygen administration during end of operative procedure to facilitate elimination of nitrous oxide.

3

Inhalational (Volatile) Anaesthetic Agents

DIETHYL ETHER

Ether is a derivative of alcohol in which H of R–O–(H) is replaced by another R group. It was first prepared by Valerius Cordus in 1546. Crawford Long in 1842 and W.T.G. Morton in 1846 first used it.

- It is colourless, pungent odour volatile liquid.
- Boiling point is 36.2°C
- It is prepared by dehydration of alcohol with sulphuric acid.
- It decomposes to acetaldehyde and peroxidase and is favored by air, light and moisture with retarded copper.
- Molecular weight is 74
- Saturated vapour pressure at 20°C is 425 mm of Hg
- Blood/gas solubility is 10 and oil/gas solubility is 3.2, MAC 1.9
- Heat of vaporization is 89 cal/gm.
- It is highly inflammable and ignites at 184°C
- The vapours are explosive when mixed with Nitrous oxide/ Oxygen.

Pharmacological actions

1. Central nervous system

- It produces irregular descending depression of central nervous

16

system. Deep tendon reflexes are exaggerated in light plane of anaesthesia. In light plane of anaesthesia, there is increased cortical and basal ganglia activity followed by central depression in deep planes.

• It produces analgesia and complete anaesthesia. It depresses the respiratory and vasomotor centers but stimulates vomiting center.

• In deep planes it produces mydriasis.

• It induces surgical anaesthesia without any premedication.

• It is safe anaesthetic agent in junior hands also but it requires some prior experience.

• It has curare-mimetic effect on skeletal muscles and produces satisfactory muscle relaxation in deep planes of anaesthesia. It potentiates the actions of non-depolarizing muscle relaxants and dose requirement of muscle relaxants is less.

• It decreases the response of respiratory center to Carbon dioxide but rate and depth of respiration is increased under Ether anaesthesia. It maintains the spontaneous respiration of the patient up to Stage III – plane II of ether anaesthesia.

• There is no change in blood pressure and does not sensitize myocardium to exogenous adrenaline so there are no any cardiac arrhythmias.

• Light planes of anaesthesia do not interfere with the uterine contractility so intermittent inhalation of ether may be recommended during labour. It crosses the placental barrier and may depress the new born.

• There is no significant liver and kidney damage with ether anaesthesia. Temporary alterations in the liver function and decrease in urine out put may be there on prolonged administration.

• It can be administered by any means of breathing system.

• It can be administered along with only air and all the time oxygen may not be necessary as it is very safe agent.

Advantages

- Margin of safety is greater than any volatile anaesthetic agent.
- It has satisfactory rapid onset of action but some what delayed than Ethyl chloride.
- It has high anaesthetic index.
- Maintenance of anaesthesia is relatively easy.
- Emergence is rapid. Reflexes and consciousness returns early but complete recovery is some what delayed.

Disadvantages

- Induction of anaesthesia is relatively slow and some times stormy, associated with excitement and retching.
- As it is irritant in nature, vapours may increase salivary and bronchial secretions and induce cough and laryngospasm during induction of anaesthesia.
- It is explosive so cautry can not be used along with it.
- Nausea and vomiting usually occurs during recovery phase. Prolonged administration may result in paralytic ileus.
- Recovery is slow so needs observations in postoperative period.
- During induction there is sensitization of baro-receptors so causes reflex inhibition of heart activity.
- Ether convulsions, ether shrucks or involuntary movements may occur postoperatively.

Indications

- For induction and maintenance of anaesthesia.
- Now a day, it is absolutely out of anaesthesia practice as better volatile agents have been introduced and are easily available.

Contraindications

- When all emergency drugs and resuscitation facilities are not available.

- Oxygen supplementation, suction apparatus and means of endotracheal intubation and ventilation facilities are not there.
- When there are no transport facilities.
- Postoperative recovery room facility with all resuscitative measures is not there.

CHLOROFORM

It was discovered in 1831 but Simpson introduced the use into clinical practice in 1847.

- It is chlorinated hydrocarbon prepared by chlorination of acetone or acetaldehyde.
- It is colourless, clear liquid with sweat odour.
- Boiling point is 61°C
- Specific gravity is 4.1205 It is non-inflammable.
- It decomposes in presence of heat and light to form aldehydes and formats. Heating causes formation of phosgene.
- It is administered by all inhalational techniques. Induction of anaesthesia requires about 4% concentration and maintenance requires 1 - 1.5% concentration. It is usually administered with oxygen.

Pharmacological Actions

Respiratory system

- It is not very irritant to respiratory tract but the secretions are produced at induction and recovery from anaesthesia.
- It increases the respiratory rate but minute ventilation is decreased.
- It produces some broncho-dilatation.

Cardiovascular system

- Cardiac rate is variable but usually decreased.
- Cardiac output is decreased by 30%.

- It is direct myocardial depressant, so various types of cardiac arrhythmias are encountered.
- It decreases peripheral vascular resistance, decreases blood pressure by reducing venous return.

Central nervous system

- There is irregular descending depression of entire central nervous system, so it is complete anaesthetic agent.
- It causes direct depression of vasomotor center.
- There is depression of respiratory, vomiting and temperature regulating centers.
- There is increase in intra-cranial pressure.

Gastro-intestinal tract

- Tone, motility and secretions of gastro-intestinal tract is decreased.
- There is marked dose dependent depression of liver functions

Genito-urinary system

- All kidney functions are decreased and anuria may be produced.
- Fatty changes in renal tubes are observed after exposure.
- There is production of metabolic acidosis due to increase in pyruvate or lactate in blood.
- Blood sugar is increased by 20%.
- There is increase in white and red blood cells.
- Oxygen content is decreased so inhibits combination of haemoglobin with oxygen and decrease affinity of oxygen to haemoglobin.
- Clotting time is decreased and capillary permeability is increased.

Advantages

- It is non-inflammable and non-irritant to mucus membrane, sweat smelling so easily accepted.

- It is most potent anaesthetic agent.
- Induction of anaesthesia is pleasant, rapid and safe.
- It has low volatility and can be used in tropical regions.
- It requires minimum equipments for administration.
- It produces excellent muscle relaxation.
- Some times can be used with only air due to low partial pressure.
- It is useful agent in short surgical procedures.

Disadvantages

- It has narrow margin of safety, so deep planes of anaesthesia are attained very quickly. With minimum obstruction hypoxia is dangerous and there are much more chances.
- It may produce dangerous hepatic toxicity
- It may cause varied degree of arrhythmias and severe myocardial depression.

ETHYL CHLORIDE

Fluorens in 1847 described the anaesthetic properties of Ethyl chloride.

- Commercially it is prepared by reaction of ethyl alcohol with hydrochloric acid.
- Boiling point is 12.5°C
- It is colourless, volatile anaesthetic agent with ethereal smell. It is slightly soluble in water and can be mixed with organic solvents.
- Molecular weight is 64.5, specific gravity is 0.92
- It is highly inflammable or forms explosive mixtures with air and oxygen.
- It should not be used in closed circuit as it is hydrolyzed by soda lime
- It is excreted unchanged by lungs.
- The agent is no more used in anaesthesia practice due to its high volatility, explosion hazards and very low margin of safety.

- It depresses the central nervous system very rapidly.
- It produces descending depression of total nervous system.
- Induction of anaesthesia as well as recovery is very fast.
- It decreases the cardiac output and directly depresses the myocardium. Initially, there is bradycardia due to vagal stimulation and then tachycardia due to ventricular fibrillation.
- Respiratory center is first stimulated then depressed.
- As it is non-irritant so do not increases the bronchial and salivary secretions but it may produce laryngospasm.
- Muscle relaxation is very less.
- It is not a safe anaesthetic agent in junior hands.
- Usually it is used for induction of anaesthesia before ether anaesthesia.
- It can be used a sole anaesthetic agent for short surgical procedures.
- It is for production of local anaesthesia due to its cooling or freezing effect on skin for incision and drainage of abscess.
- It is not recommended for prolonged use.
- It is contraindicated in patients with pre-existing cardiac arrhythmias, myocardial diseases and conduction defects.
- It is also contraindicated in severe liver and kidney diseases.

TRICHLOROETHYLENE – Trilene

Trilene was discovered by Fisher in 1864 and since then used in industry for dye cleaning as it is fat solvent or to remove grease.

Anaesthetic properties were described by Lehmann in 1911 and D Jackson popularized in anaesthesia in 1933.

Now a days, the used is banned due to fear of toxicity and availability of newer, safe and potent inhalational anaesthetic agents.

- It is clear colourless volatile agent with sweat smell.
- Molecular weight is 131
- Boiling point is 86°C
- Specific gravity is 1.47
- Oil/water solubility is 400, blood/gas solubility 9

- Saturated vapour pressure is 60 mm of Hg
- Vapour density 4.35 and MAC is 0.17
- It is stable and decomposed in light, air and heat.
- It contains0.01% thymol as preservative and waxolline blue to colour the drug for identification as it is similar to chloroform.
- It is not explosive or inflammable
- Exposure of Trilene to air or sunlight causes oxidation to produce dichloroacetyl chloride, carbon monoxide, hydrochloric acid and phosgene.
- Soda lime decomposes it into dichloroacetylene, which is very toxic and causes nerve palsies and phosgene in presence of heat.
- It is relatively soluble in blood so induction of anaesthesia and recovery is delayed. High lipid solubility gives it high potency but due to low saturated vapour pressure produces difficulty to achieve the appropriate concentration.
- It is powerful analgesic and good general anaesthetic agent. There is overall central nervous system depression with sedation and amnesia.
- Induction of anaesthesia is smooth but takes some time and so also recovery is delayed.
- There are no excessive salivary and bronchial secretions.
- There is no alteration in liver and kidney functions.
- It produces very poor skeletal muscle relaxation.
- There is no increase in metabolic rate.
- It rapidly crosses the placental barrier and adequate concentration is reached in the foetal circulation.
- In low concentration it does not interfere with progress of labour but in high concentrations, it depresses myometrial contractions.
- There is no change in blood pressure but it results in various types of arrhythmias. It may cause bradycardia due to vagal stimulation or deep planes may cause extra systoles, bigemini

or tachycardia. These arrhythmias are usually due to hypoxia, hypercarbia or increased levels of catecholamines.

- It produces tachypnoea in deeper planes of anaesthesia. It stimulates and sensitizes the deflation receptors and so causes rapid and shallow respiration leading to hypoxia and hypercarbia.
- Mostly it is excreted unchanged via lungs. 20–30% is broken down in liver to Trichloroethanol and trichloroacetic acid. The metabolic products may remain in the body for 10–13 days.

Indications

- As it is potent analgesic, so it is recommended during labour, minor urological procedures, change of dressings, short surgical procedures, dental analgesia.
- Postoperative pain relief.
- As analgesic in balanced technique of anaesthesia.

Contraindications

- Severe cardiac disease
- Cardiac failure either left ventricular or congestive cardiac failure
- Toxemia of pregnancy
- When the use of Adrenaline is indicated.
- In presence of closed circuit.

Adverse effects

- It produces variety of cardiac arrhythmias from bradycardia to ventricular tachycardia or fibrillation.
- Severe tachypnoea, which may interfere in normal respiration and may lead to hypoxia or hypercarbia.
- It sensitizes myocardium to exogenous catecholamines.
- It reacts with soda lime to produce trichloroethylene into dichloroacetylene and neurotoxin.

- It results in dangerous cranial nerve palsy or trigeminal neuralgia.
- Now a day it is no more used.

HALOTHANE

Halothane was first prepared by Suckling in 1951 and Johnstone first time used clinically in 1956. It is halogenated fluorocarbon.

- It is colourless volatile anaesthetic agent with characteristic sweet smell.
- Molecular weight is 197.4
- Boiling point is 50°C
- Latent heat of vaporization is 35.2°C
- Saturated vapour pressure at 20°C is 243 mm of Hg
- Specific gravity is 1.87
- Oil/water solubility is 220, blood/gas solubility is 2.5 and MAC is 0.2
- It is stored in amber coloured bottles as it is decomposed by light. It contains 0.01% thymol as preservative.
- It is not explosive and not inflammable.
- It can be used along with soda lime in closed circuit and some portion is absorbed in rubber.
- It is potent anaesthetic agent.
- It causes smooth descending depression of central nervous system. It causes dose and concentration dependent depression of almost all centers in the central nervous system.
- Pharyngeal and laryngeal reflexes are depressed so one can intubate the patient under halothane anaesthesia.
- It increases cerebral blood flow there by increases intra-cranial pressure.
- It causes dose dependent respiratory and vasomotor center depression. There is more depression of sympathetic system as compared to parasympathetic nervous system.
- It decreases cardiac output, stroke volume, arterial pressure and myocardial contractility by direct action on heart. Systemic

vascular resistance is not altered. Hypotension is due to decrease in cardiac output.

• Myocardial oxygen demand is decreased as there is reduction in myocardial contractility, heart rate, left ventricular wall tension and cardiac work. So bradycardia and Hypotension are common under halothane anaesthesia.

• Ventricular automaticity is depressed. It sensitizes myocardium for exogenous catecholamines and so varied arrhythmias are encountered.

• It directly depresses vascular smooth muscles to cause vasodilatation and thus protects the patient from shock syndrome.

• It is not irritating to respiratory tract so does not increase salivary and tracheo-bronchial secretions. it reduces the tidal volume and increases the respiratory rate resulting in diminished alveolar ventilation. There are chances of hypoxia under halothane anaesthesia so respiration should be controlled or assisted. It produces some broncho-dilatation.

• It itself produces some muscle relaxation and potentiates the actions of depolarizing and non-depolarizing muscle relaxants.

• It does not affect normal renal functions.

• It causes hypersensitive type hepato-toxicity after its administration. Microscopically it causes fatal lesions like viral hepatitis. Recently it is claimed to be non-hepato toxic but liver damage may occur with intermediate hepato-toxic metabolites produced in a reductive metabolic pathway of halothane. The reductive pathway is stimulated by hypoxia.

• It crosses placental barrier but at 2–3% concentrations it inhibits active uterine contractions and also may lead to post-partum haemorrhage. In concentrations less than 0.5% it reduces the incidence of awareness during caesarian section. Foetal concentration is very less.

• Postoperative nausea and vomiting is less after halothane anaesthesia.

• Post-anaesthesiae is most commonly observed as there is peripheral vasodilatation and Hypotension.

- The recovery from anaesthesia is rapid after the stoppage of drug administration.
- It may exaggerate the clinical features of malignant hyper pyrexia or it may trigger the response.
- Mostly it is excreted unchanged by the lungs and partly about 20% is metabolized in the liver into the metabolites as bromine, chlorine, trifluoro acetic acid and trifluoro ethanol amide.
- The metabolites and halothane are blamed to be hepato toxic.
- It can be administered by open drop, semi-open, semi-closed or in closed circuit. During open drop method, the wastage is more and the expenditure encored will be too much as it is costly.
- Fluotec Mark II or Mark III vaporizer is used for economical purpose as it gives measured concentration of halothane. It was previously administered via Goldman vaporizer but the concentration cannot be increased beyond 2%.

Advantages

- Non-inflammable
- Rapid and smooth induction of anaesthesia with rapid recovery.
- It is potent so recommended for complete anaesthesia.
- Non-irritating and sweet smelling so accepted by paediatric patients and there are no salivary and tracheal secretions.
- Smooth muscle and uterine relaxant.
- In low concentration it is cardiostable

Disadvantages

- In high concentrations it is effective myocardial depressant and results into severe systemic hypotension.
- There are chances of bradycardia due myocardial depression and tachycardia due systemic hypotension.
- Dose and concentration dependent liver damage postoperatively.
- There are chances of post-partum haemorhage.

Indications

- For induction and maintenance of anaesthesia in critically ill patients.
- For short surgical procedures as a sole anaesthetic agent.
- As an adjuvant to balanced technique of anaesthesia.
- As supplementation to regional anaesthesia.
- For production of deliberate hypotension in indicated operative procedures and in some patients.
- For endotracheal intubation where there is anticipated difficult intubation or for blind nasal intubation.
- As a smooth muscle relaxant particularly manual removal of placenta.
- In extremes of age group due to its high potency.

Contraindications

- Recent myocardial infarction or insufficiency
- Recent congestive cardiac failure or digitalization
- In severe shock patients due to any cause.
- Known case of liver diseases
- Routine obstetrics.

Now a day, newer inhalational anaesthetic agents have been introduced in anaesthesia practice so old ones are discarded and are also not available. The new ones are Enflurane, Isoflurane, Sevoflurane, Fluroxene, Desflurane, etc are under trial and some of them are in use. Out of these Isoflurane and Sevoflurane are well practiced due to their high potency, easy acceptability, cardiovascular stability, and alternative pathway of elimination as Hoffmann degradation, less hepato toxicity.

The only problem with these drugs is that, these are very costly and so in government hospitals are not affordable. These require special vaporizer for vaporization, which is also costly.

4

Preoperative Assessment and Preparation

Every patient posted for major or minor operative procedures under any anaesthesia (even local anesthesia) should be evaluated by expert anaesthesiologist for fitness of anaesthesia and surgery. A patient posted for minor operative procedure under local anaesthesia may require supplementation in the form of sedation, sedation with analgesia or general anaesthesia for the completion of surgery.

At this occasion, it is better that the patient should have been preoperatively evaluated for fitness of anaesthesia to avoid complications related to anaesthesia. So every patient posted for any operative procedure under any anaesthesia should be evaluated for fitness of anaesthesia by expert anaesthesiologists as far the one who is going to administer anaesthesia to the patient.

Aims of Preoperative Evaluation

- Introduction of anaesthesiologist (himself) to the patient about his role during operative procedure.
- To allay anxiety, fear in the patients for operation and particularly anaesthesia
- To detect associated medical disorders of various systems related to the conduction of anaesthesia and perioperative correlation by asking the history of these disorders of various systems.

- After detection and confirmation of diagnosis, these patients are referred to experts of various fraternities and these are advised to take treatment for it to optimize the physical status for smooth conduction of anaesthesia with minimum perioperative complications.

- To advice for the drug therapy which these patients might be receiving for the systemic disorders. In this regard one should advice for which drugs should be continued on the day of operation or which drugs should be omitted on the day of operation for smooth conduction of anaesthesia. This is important in relation to drug interaction of these drugs with various drugs used during administration of anaesthesia technique.

- To advice for relevant and important investigations for confirmation of associated medical disorder and also to see progress of disease.

- To emphasize the importance of nil by mouth at least 4–6 hours before scheduled time of operative to avoid perioperative chances of vomiting and regurgitation.

- Main aim of preoperative evaluation is to avoid un-necessary postponement of operation and to provide better quality-oriented anaesthesia to minimize perioperative morbidity and mortality.

OBJECTIVES OF PREOPERATIVE EVALUATION

- To provide better quality of anaesthesia to every patient.

- To minimize perioperative complications related to drugs used during conduct of anaesthesia, technique of anaesthesia and to provide optimum conditions for completion of operative procedure.

- To administer desirable technique of anaesthesia to every patient posted for operative procedure which might be minor or major.

- To avoid un-necessary postponement of patient for minor technical or medical problems, which are ultimately cost beneficial for patient and as well as for the government. This can be accomplished by changing the technique of anaesthesia.

- To provide acceptable technique of anaesthesia to the patient and to surgeon.

PREOPERATIVE EVALUATION

- One should see the case paper of the patient for identification, detail case notes, provisional diagnosis, treatment, physical status of the patient in relation to progress of disease or effect of therapy, investigations, referral to experts and operative procedure planned.

- One must see the previous operative procedure if carried out in the same patient, technique of anaesthesia received and whether there were any problems during conduction of anaesthesia perioperatively.

- **Sex :** It is important to note the sex of patient as some diseases are common in some sex. The surgical pathology may be different in male or female patients or common in both. Detail obstetric history should be evaluated in female patients as when the patient is in carrying state then any elective operative procedure is contraindicated. In male patients history of addiction should be asked as these are prone for it.

- **Age :** Noting down age of the patient is very important in relation to various surgical pathologies are particularly common in certain age groups. There are some physiological differences in paediatric and geriatric patients as compared to adult patients. So one has to be very particular during preanaesthesia evaluations and accordingly examine these patients. Age is also important for taking valid written consent for anaesthesia and surgery. In these aspects age has importance during preanaesthesia evaluation of patients.

- **History taking :** In every patient related history according to age of the patient, sex of patient and surgical pathology with ruling out of any associated, undiagnosed medical disorder, drug therapy should be asked and patient should be clinically evaluated accordingly.

- All patients should be asked questions to rule out association of individual system disorders –

1. Respiratory system

a) History of cough

- Whether present or not, if present then
- Whether cough is with sputum or dry one
- What is colour of sputum – white, yellowish gray, blood
- What is amount of sputum (quantity) less or more
- Whether foul smelling or not
- Whether tinge of blood or frank haemoptasis
- Any postural relation
- Any aggravating or relieving factors

b) Whether there is history of breathlessness

- Whether it is progressive
- Whether difficulty in respiration is during expiration or inspiration (lower airway obstruction or upper airway obstruction)
- Whether known case of Bronchial asthma. If yes, then one must ask for the treatment history, aggravating and relieving factors, seasonal variations, allergy to any drugs or environmental conditions,etc
- One must ask history of chest pain and its relation to the respiratory cycle. One must differentiate it from myocardial chest pain. The site of chest pain should be located and whether it is referred or not. Whether chest pain has any postural relation or any aggravating or relieving factors.
- One must ask history of oedema over feet, epigastric discomfort, breathlessness to rule out possibility of congestive cardiac failure secondary to chronic obstructive airway disease. It should be differentiated from CCF due to cardiac disease, liver, kidney involvement or anaemia hypoproteinaemia.
- One must ask for occupation of the patient to rule out

association of pulmonary diseases related to occupational hazards like pneumoconiosis.

- One must ask history of fever to rule out possibility of pulmonary infection acute or chronic in origin. Whether fever is high grade or low grade, whether associated with chills and rigors. One must ask history of upper respiratory tract infection as change in voice, pharyngeal irritation, rhinórrhoea, etc.
- One must ask history of aspiration pneumonitis as history of unconsciousness, alcoholism, etc. The history of chronic amoebiasis should be ruled out.
- One must ask history of smoking as the pulmonary diseases are most common in these peoples and if yes one must ask for quantity and if stopped then from how many days should be enquired.
- One must ask history of repeated attacks of cyanosis and should be differentiated from congenital heart diseases.

2. Cardiovascular diseases

a. Breathlessness

- It may be due to congestive cardiac failure secondary to right sided obstructive pathology, left ventricular failure, fixed low cardiac output states or severe hypertension, etc.
- It should be differentiated from congestive cardiac failure due chronic obstructive airway diseases, liver, kidney, hypoproteinemia or due to pregnancy.
- Breathlessness may be due to severe anaemia.
- This breathlessness is always associated with paroxysmal nocturnal dyspnoea.

b. Palpitation

It is unpleasant awareness of own heart beats. It may be idiopathic or secondary to anxiety, fear, hyper dynamic circulation (anaemia, thyrotoxicosis, pregnancy, exercise, tea, coffee), ischemic heart disease, hypertensive heart disease, rheumatic heart disease, myopathies or left ventricular failure, congestive cardiac failure, etc. It denotes organic heart disease.

c. Cough

Here cough should be differentiated from respiratory pathology. Cough in heart diseases is due to pulmonary involvement. Usually it is due to congestive cardiac failure secondary to any cause and it is dry type or with scanty or watery sputum. In pulmonary hypertension and left ventricular failure also watery sputum is observed.

The cough with mucoid sputum or frothy sputum is always presenting cardiac pathology. Frank haemoptasis is there in Mitral stenosis and pulmonary embolism.

d. Chest pain

One must ask history of chest pain which is usually sudden in onset with some precipitating factors. It is intense, intolerable, retro-sternal, referred to left shoulder and medial side of arm. This chest pain should be differentiated from the chest pain of respiratory origin, which is related to respiratory cycle, or costo-chondral origin.

When history of chest pain due to ischemic heart disease is positive, then one must keep in mind that elective operative procedures are contraindicated for a period of at least 6 months. One has take special intensive care during emergency operative procedures in these patients of ischemic heart disease.

e. Headache

History of headache should be asked to rule out possibility of hypertensive heart disease. Some times headache is associated with vision disturbances. Headache should be differentiated from common causes as upper respiratory tract infection or uncommon causes as raised intra-cranial tension, space occupying lesions, glaucoma, migraine, etc.

f. Syncope attacks

It should be asked to rule out possibility of low fixed cardiac output states or severe anaemia.

g. Oedema over feet

It should be asked to rule out congestive cardiac failure due to right-sided obstructive pathology or other causes as pulmonary disease, liver, kidney or hypoproteinemia states.

3. Central nervous system

To rule out central nervous system involvement, one must ask history of headache, convulsions, vertigo, sensory loss, loss of motor power in any group of muscles, involuntary movements, generalized weakness, unconsciousness, head injury, myopathies, etc. This is to confirm the extent of neurological deficit and one must take care that the existing neurological sequels should not be exaggerated due to technique of anaesthesia. Care should be taken during administration of general as well as regional technique of anaesthesia.

4. Liver

To rule out the possibility of liver involvement one must ask history of jaundice (yellow discolouration of conjunctiva, skin or urine), epigastric discomfort, nausea, vomiting, oedema over feet, alcohol addiction, bleeding tendency, serum hepatitis, blood transfusion, hepato-toxic drugs, previous anaesthetic exposure with halothane, prolonged or delayed recovery from anaesthesia, etc.

This all is important as many of the drugs used during perioperative period are metabolized in liver and if liver functions are already impoured then there is possibility of prolonged effects of these drugs or there might be exaggeration of liver damage and some there are chances of morbidity and mortality perioperatively.

5. Gastro-intestinal tract

The involvement of gastro-intestinal tract does not affect the course of anaesthesia directly. In these patients with history of vomiting, diarrhoea or fluid loss due to any reasons, there are chances of electrolyte and acid base in balance which indirectly affects the course of general anaesthesia. Electrolyte balance is important in relation to cardiac functions, excretion of drugs, neuromuscular transmission and fluid balance perioperatively. Fluid and electrolyte imbalance is important in various oedema states and affects the out come of patients.

6. Renal system

One must ask urine out put, burning in micturation, history of renal or ureteric colic, and oedema over feet, etc. to assess the renal functions. This is important in relation that most of the drugs used during perioperative period are excreted via kidneys and its functions should be normal otherwise there might be delayed recovery from anaesthesia or drug adverse effects. These are important in relation to administration of intravenous fluids. It is more important during emergency operative procedures.

7. Endocrine disorders

One must ask history to rule out possibility of Diabetes mellitus, Thyroid gland dysfunctions, Addison's disease, Hyper-aldestorism, pheochromocytoma or congenital diseases.. In these diseases one has to ask for treatment history and progress of disease and has to take due precautions during conduction of anaesthesia.

8. Miscellaneous history

One must ask history of major illness in the past, treatment received for the same and change in physical status so that due precautions or alterations in the conduction of anaesthesia can be taken. This is applicable to all systemic diseases.

One must ask history of addiction in young and adult patients particularly of smoking, tobacco chewing, alcohol or any other so that alterations or its ill effects on body can be assessed and due precautions during conduction of anaesthesia can be taken.

In male patients it is important to ask the history of smoking (cigarette or bidi), duration, quantity and whether stopped or not. It is related to presence of cardiovascular or respiratory system disorders.

History of alcohol consumption is important in relation to liver dysfunction or head injury or other multiple injuries and aspiration pneumonitis.

One must ask history of previous operative procedure and technique of anaesthesia so that if there were any problems during that event then one can take precautions to avoid those problems during present operative procedure. This is important to reduce chances of morbidity and mortality related to technique of anaesthesia.

One must enquire about the technique of anaesthesia adopted in previous operative procedures as repeated regional blocks, halothane exposure so that these can be avoided by changing the technique of anaesthesia.

One history of drug sensitivity or anaphylactic reactions, which can be avoided, or precautions can be taken as induction agents, narcotic analgesics or muscle relaxants and intravenous fluids.

In female patients one must ask history of last menstrual cycle as elective operative procedures are relatively contraindicated during this period. This is also true for first or last trimester of pregnancy.

One must enquire about drug therapy for respiratory, cardiovascular, endocrinal, neuro-muscular, haematological, nutritional, occupational disorders as some drugs should be discontinued or some should continued on the day of operative procedure to avoid chances of drug interactions and smooth conduction of anaesthesia.

The age and sex of the patient is many times obvious but it should be confirmed as some medical disorders are common in particular age group or there might be physiological or anatomical differences is some age group (paediatric & geriatric). This is also important in relation in obtaining valid consent for anaesthesia and surgery.

Particularly during emergency operative procedures, the timing of last meal should be asked as the patients are usually asked to be nil by mouth at least for 6–8 hours for elective operations. During all emergency operations as far as possible all patients should be considered to be with full stomach (Orthopaedic procedures, caesarian section, upper abdominal operations or obstruction.

Trauma) as pain may be contributing factor for delaying emptying time of stomach. Here due precautions should be taken to avoid chances of vomiting and aspiration during induction of general anaesthesia.

During emergency procedures one must enquire about voiding of urine or confirm urine output in the patients which indicates status of hydration, kidney functions and circulatory status particularly in trauma patients, gastro-intestinal obstruction, perforation peritonitis, etc. It is important during administration of which are totally excreted via kidney and intravenous fluid administration, this intern affects total outcome of patients.

GENERAL EXAMINATION

These patients should be examined in detail to correlate the medical disorders or normal variations and surgical pathology.

One must see for consciousness of patient which is important only during emergency procedures and not usually in elective patients. Whether patient is conscious, semi-conscious or unconscious due to various medical disorders of central nervous system or as late manifestations of cardiovascular, respiratory, endocrinal, hepatic, renal, metabolic disorders. The change in consciousness may due to head injury or haemorrhagic shock.

When the patient is unconscious or semiconscious then general anaesthesia is not required and one must monitor vital signs and the procedure can be performed under local anaesthesia with regional blocks or only sedation.

One must see the built of the patient as – well built, moderate, obese, malnourished or cachexic. This is important in relation to dosage of drugs, fluid and electrolyte balance, regional anaesthesia and recovery of the patient. One must be careful in very cachexic and morbidly obese patients as there might be associated medical disorders. Obese patients may prose problems during positioning and regional blocks.

One must confirm that whether the patient is cooperative or not which is necessary during regional blocks and spinal, epidural blocks. This indicated that patients might be having psychological or metabolic and central nervous system disturbances. These patients may be on therapy for these problems and mainly anti-psychotic drugs may have drug interaction with inducing agents, narcotic analgesics and sedatives. Paediatric and geriatric patients and chronically ill patients are not cooperative.

One must see, whether patient is comfortable in bed or not. Uncomfortable patient might have acute pain due to any cause, upper or lower respiratory distress, urinary retention or psychological disturbances. One should see that the patient should be comfortable before evaluation as well as before induction of anaesthesia by relieving the causative factor.

One must see whether patient is febrile or not. When patient is not febrile then there is no problem. When febrile, the elevated ten.perature should be brought down before induction of anaesthesia. Here one should keep in mind that, elevated temperature pose the problems as increase in requirement of Oxygen, intravenous fluids, there might be more fluid loss, dehydration, decrease in urine output, there is contraindication for use of Atropine sulphate and Suxamethonium, chances of convulsions, hyperpyrexia, left ventricular failure, etc.

To avoid these perioperative problems the temperature of the patient should be brought down before induction of anaesthesia. It is indicative of definite infection in the body. As far as possible active infection should be controlled before elective operations and due precautions should be taken in emergency situations with preloading by antibiotics or cooling of body, etc.

- Pulse of the patient should be seen for palpability, rate, rhythm, volume and equality on both sides. All these features of the pulse are very important as for monitoring of patient, administration of drugs, intravenous fluids, cardiovascular alterations, peripheral circulation and other perioperative complications. Preoperative assessment of pulse is important as immediate resuscitation requirement before induction of anaesthesia, technique of anaesthesia, choice of drugs, inducing agents, muscle relaxants, intravenous fluid administration, Ventilatory pattern and avoidance of related complications.

Changes in pulse rate, rhythm, volume are indicative of either cardiovascular, myocardial or peripheral circulatory disorders. Pulse alterations may be observed as effect of other disorders as respiratory system, late stages of severe hepatic or renal disorders, endocrinal, trauma, pain, electrolyte and fluid imbalance, active infection in the body, anxiety, etc. What ever the cause of alterations in pulse parameters are there it should well diagnosed and treated accordingly and due care should be taken during conduction of anaesthesia.

- **Blood Pressure :** Preoperative blood pressure with desirable size of cuff in various age groups should be noted as basal reading. When systolic and diastolic blood pressure for that age group is normal then there is no problem. When higher or lower systolic and diastolic blood pressure are obtained, then it should be confirmed with ruling out normal physiological variations.

  When hypotension is noted which is encountered during emergency operations which might be due to haemorhagic shock or any other type of shock states, hypovolumia, the exact cause should be seen and treated accordingly to optimize the blood pressure before induction of anaesthesia. When hypertension is noted then should be confirmed by repeated readings and treated accordingly before induction of anaesthesia.

  Hypotension or hypertension should be well treated so that direct effects of sedatives, narcotic analgesics, intravenous induction agents, inhalational anaesthetic agents, muscle relaxants, ventilation pattern, technique of anaesthesia, blood loss during operations, anaphylaxis, etc, will have minimum effects in terms of morbidity and mortality related to changes in blood pressure during conduction of anaesthesia.

- One should see that whether patient is pale or not. Pallor indicate the status of anaemia or blood volume in the patient which is important during preoperative preparation of the patient, fitness for anaesthesia and surgery, expected blood loss during operation and its effects on the total out come of the patient in terms of morbidity and mortality. So when the patient is moderate to severe pale one should confirm the exact cause of anaemia and blood loss, whether acute or chronic in origin, necessity of perioperative blood transfusion, blood reservation and technique of anaesthesia. Pallor is commonly seen on the conjunctiva, tongue or nail bed.

- Then one must see whether there is ictrus or jaundice present or not. When ictrus is present, it is definite indicative of liver dysfunction and it is stated that, elective operative procedures are absolutely contraindicated minimum for 6 months to avoid morbidity and mortality. Noting liver functions is important as all anaesthesia drugs as sedatives, narcotic analgesics, muscle relaxants and inhalational anaesthetic agents are metabolized in liver, clotting mechanism may be altered in presence of liver disturbances. The deepness of jaundice also indicates the cause of liver dysfunction and is beneficial in diagnosis and treatment. Only obstructive jaundice are accepted in presence of deep jaundice as these patients are posted for removal of cause.

- Baldness of scalp is many times familiar or noted in old age but at an early age is may be indicative of cirrhosis of liver.

- Loss of hairs of eye brow may be cosmetic in female but it is diagnostic of Hanson's disease, there may be peripheral neuropathy, paraesthesia patches and postural hypotension.

- Sunken or dragged eyes are diagnostic of dehydration due to gastro-intestinal disturbances noted easily in paediatric patients.

- Squint is diagnostic of neuro-muscular disorders, nystagmus may be hereditary or associated with neuro-muscular disease.

- Depressed bridge of nose may be racial or familial, old fracture of nose and may prose problems during nasal intubation. So one must see patency of both nostrils when nasal intubation is indicated.

- Oral cavity should be inspected for loose teeth, absence of teeth, artificial denture, bleeding gums, size of tongue, any intra-oral growth, evidence of fracture of mandible or maxilla, to rule out possibility of difficult laryngoscopy and intubation.

- One must see neck movements and movements at temporo-mandibular joint for laryngoscopy and endotracheal intubation.
- Colour of tongue is noted for paleness or smoothness, which is indicative status of anaemia. In turn it is important for preoperative blood transfusion requirement.
- Upper airway is inspected for congestion, secretions, obstruction, pharynx or larynx to rule out presence of infection as it is contraindicated for fitness of anaesthesia. Here there are chances of infection to travel down lower airway and bronchospasm or laryngospasm. During nasal intubation there are chances of profuse bleeding.
- One should see whether jugular venous pressure is normal, raised or low. Raised JVP indicates obstruction to venous flow or congestive cardiac failure either due to cardiovascular, respiratory, hepatic, renal or haemopoetic pathology. Bilaterally raised JVP indicates obstruction at thoracic inlet. Low JVP indicates moderate to severe hypovolumia due to any cause. The patients with raised JVP mainly due to congestive cardiac failure are not fit for elective operative procedures. Low JVP patients are preoperatively resuscitated before induction of anaesthesia.
- Cervical lymphadenopathy should be excluded indicative upper respiratory tract infection or neoplastic and blood cell or lymphatic cell disorders which is not so important during elective operations. Here it indicates chronic medical disorder, which should be thoroughly investigated and treated accordingly.
- Neck movements as flexion, extension and side to side movements should be confirmed when general anaesthesia with endotracheal intubation is planned. It should be particularly seen in patients with anticipated difficult laryngoscopy and intubation. The neck movements may be restricted in cervical vertebral abnormality, swelling in front or back of neck and some one has to change the technique of anaesthesia.
- Puffiness of face usually indicates severe congestive cardiac failure due to any cause or pre-eclamptic toxemia. There may

be generalized accumulation fluid in the extra-vascular compartment. It poses problems during laryngoscopy, endotracheal intubation, fluid calculation and intravenous administration, calculation of doses of drugs according to weight and access of veins.

• Clubbing of fingers indicates chronic state of disease which may be due to respiratory pathology (Suppurative lung disease), cardiovascular (congenital heart disease), gastro-intestinal (malabsorption syndrome), liver or endocrinal disorders. It does not directly influence course of anaesthesia but these patients should be thoroughly investigated for causative factor and treated accordingly be fore induction of anaesthesia.

• Cyanosis is the bluish tinge or discolouration of mucosa or nail beds which may be peripheral or central and acute or chronic in origin. It is due to increased amount of reduced haemoglobin (more than 5 gm%) in capillary bed. Peripheral cyanosis occurs due to stasis of blood or delayed oxygen supply to tissues. Central cyanosis is due to diminished arterial oxygen saturation. Peripheral cyanosis is due to respiratory obstruction and central cyanosis is due to cardiovascular disorders. Any cyanosis is medical emergency and causative facture should be eliminated before induction of anaesthesia. In these patients there are every chances of development of cyanosis any time perioperatively and should take care to treat it avoid recurrence.

• Oedema over feet should be elicited for its presence, pitting or non-pitting, unilateral or bilateral. Oedema over feet may be minimal or severe according to severity of disease, It may be due to congestive cardiac failure secondary to respiratory, cardiovascular, renal, hepatic, myxoedema, anaemia with hypoproteinemia, pre-eclampsia and gastro-intestinal disorders which should be investigated and treated accordingly before operations and anaesthesia. The presence of oedema over feet and body, poses problems due weight gain, drug dose calculations, intravenous fluid infusion, electrolyte balance, excretion of drugs and even taking venous access and shifting of patient.

- Built of the patient as gigantism, dwarfism, should be noted and related changes in anaesthesia technique or precautions should be kept in mind.
- Vertebral column should be seen as it is important during induction of spinal epidural blocks, positioning of patient. In severe abnormalities as kyphosis, scoliosis and lordosis, it has associated restrictive airway disease and chances of postoperative complications related to respiratory system.
- Rarely thickened nerves are noted as in Hansen's disease and other neuromuscular disorders which are of importance during regional anaesthesia.
- Skin of the patient should be seen for colour, pigmentation, eruptions, patecheal haemorhage, nails, hairs, etc. which are of less importance as far as technique of anaesthesia but should be noted.
- Respiration of the patient should be observed and its importance is only during emergency operative procedures preoperatively and after anaesthesia postoperatively. Any abnormalities of the respiration in elective or emergency patients should be corrected as far as possible before induction of anaesthesia. During emergency, one should confirm that patient is not in the respiratory arrest. The respiration should be seen for rate, type, regularity, change in pattern, cyanosis, etc.

  Then one should look for whether, there is upper or lower respiratory tract obstruction resulting difficulty in respiration, centrally originated tachypnoea, restrictive or obstructive airway disease, inadequate respiration and cynosis, signs of hypoxia, breath holding, etc. All these features should be seen, treated accordingly in view of adequate oxygenation. The respiration parameters may be altered due to respiratory pathology or terminal events of chronic disease. The patient should be well oxygenated, settled for abnormality and then accepted for operative procedure under anaesthesia. As far as in these patients regional techniques should be preferred over general anaesthesia and use of sedatives and narcotic analgesics should be avoided.

SYSTEMIC EXAMINATION

During systemic examination, according to relevant positive points in history and general examination, the systemic examination should be carried of the system first and in detail, which is affected most, and other systems should be examined as usual in detail. The systemic examination should be aimed in accordance with technique of anaesthesia to be adopted or which is safe in that patient, drug metabolism used perioperatively and minimum morbidity and mortality related to conduction of anaesthesia and operative procedure.

Central nervous system

One should see for

- Consciousness
- Hearing in old age
- Vision – old age and hypertensive and diabetic patients
- Cooperation – psychologically disturbed patients, old and paediatric patients
- Orientation in time and place – in patients with head injury, cerebro-vascular accidents, under effect of sedatives and alcoholics, etc.
- Motor power – in patients with head injury, neuro-muscular disorders, electrolyte imbalance, critically ill patients, etc.
- Sensory system – for pain, touch, temperature in patients with motor neuron disease.
- Reflexes – all tendon reflexes, laryngeal, pharyngeal, gag reflex in central nervous system disorders or in head injury.

Consciousness is very important for the induction of anaesthesia. When the patient is fully conscious then there is no problem. Semiconscious patients may have associated head injury, hypoxia, hypovolumia, haemorhagic shock, severe electrolyte imbalance, renal or hepatic failure, etc. Here only sedation or local anaesthesia is sufficient to carry out operations. Unconsciousness may be due to severe systemic disease particularly of respiratory, cardiovascular, hepatic or renal disease or may be terminal stage of life. Here, there is no necessary of any anaesthesia and only vital parameters should be monitored continuously.

2. Respiratory system

Here patients should be examined for presence of respiration, rate, rhythm, regularity, adequacy and type.

Inspection

One should carry out inspection for :
- symmetry of chest,
- bilateral movements,
- position of trachea,
- retraction or bulging,
- visible veins over chest wall,
- sinuses, puncture marks,
- position of ribs (horizontal or normal),
- any congenital abnormalities of rib cage, etc.

These all should be clinically correlated..

Palpation

All inspectory findings should be confirmed by palpation as :
- position of trachea (deviation to one side),
- respiratory movements,
- tenderness,
- apical impulse in relation to respiratory pathology,
- tactile vocal fremitus,
- palpable respiratory sounds, etc.

Percussion

All areas of chest wall should be percussed. One should note that :
- whether percussion note is normal or changed,

- whether it is impaired – resonant, tympanic, dull, stony dull,
- upper border of liver dullness,
- cardiac dullness,
- tenderness over chest wall,
- shifting dullness, etc.

Auscultation

- Presence of air entry – present or completely absent
- Air entry whether adequate or inadequate
- Whether present in all areas and up to bases
- Normal as vesicular or bronchial type
- Added sounds as crepitations (fine or course, bubbling), Rhonchi, rales. Pleural rub, intestinal sounds.
- Quality of heart sounds.

3. Cardiovascular system

Cardiovascular system should be examined as :

a. Inspection

- Precordium – Normal or bulging
- Apical impulse – Visible or not, position, any shift
- Visible Pulsations over precordial area, epigastric, supraclavicular, etc.
- Venous engorgement
- Jugular venous pressure

b. Palpation

- Confirmation of apex beat
- Whether normal, changed in character, shifted or not
- Palpable murmur called as thrill in all four areas of heart
- Palpation in II intercostal space for diastolic shock
- Parasternal heave – right or left to note ventricular hypertrophy

- Confirmation of pulsation in epigastric, supraclavicular areas
- Tenderness over Precordium

c. Percussion

Percussion should be carried out to note cardiac dullness with its boundaries – left heart border, right heart border, epigastric dullness, dull note in second intercostals space, liver dullness on right side.

d. Auscultation

- For confirmation of heart sounds for presence, quality – muffled at Mitral area
- To differentiate between first and second heart sounds
- Gap in between two heart sound, normal or prolonged, whether associated with any murmur, type of murmur, whether systolic or diastolic, localization, radiation, intensity, opening snap, presystolic extuations.
- Heart sounds should be noted in Mitral, Tricuspid, Pulmonary and Aortic areas for all characters.
- One should note presence of gallop or III heart sound, precordial rub
- Any variations in heart sounds should be correlated with association of respiratory system disorders or intra-thoracic abnormalities.

4. Gastro-intestinal system

- Examination of gastro-intestinal system is not so important as far as technique of anaesthesia is concerned. Only inspection is relatively important.
- On inspection large abdominal belly or obesity will prose problems during supine position as well as during prone and lateral positions. It creates problem during spontaneous breathing while regional anaesthesia or respiratory inadequacy post-operatively.
- Scaphoid shape of abdomen (empty abdomen) indicates all

abdominal contents in the thoracic cavity or indicative of diaphragmatic or ventral hernia.

- Paralytic ileus indicates electrolyte imbalance which should be corrected before induction of anaesthesia
- Free fluid or ascitis indicates congestive cardiac failure due to any cause.

5. Endocrinal system

Endocrinal disorders are usually evident on general examination or other systemic involvement can be detected on systemic examination. Mild endocrinal involvement should be suspected and diagnosed after investigations and treated accordingly.

6. Neuromuscular system

One should see over all muscles which indicate built of patient and is important during dosage of drugs and intravenous fluids. Less muscle correlates with chronic illness, cachexia, malignancy, malnourishment, muscle dystrophy, Juvenile diabetes, etc.

Good muscle mass with weakness indicate myopathies and neuro-muscular disorders which affects administration and metabolism of muscle relaxants.

- Infection of various joints or arthritis prose problem during positioning of patients.

- Geriatric and paediatric patients should be seen carefully along with relatives or parents for good feedback. These patients differ in various aspects which correlate as far as conduction of anaesthesia is concerned.

- Then one must come to a provisional diagnosis of associated medical disorder may be affecting or not affecting surgical pathology or which might be secondary to surgical pathology. The diagnosis should be confirmed on clinical findings as well as with aid of related investigations.

- In these patients routine should asked to carry out which are of prime importance for conduction of anaesthesia and special investigations should be asked in indicated patients for ease of administration of anaesthesia.

Routine Investigations

1. Haemoglobin estimation

Haemoglobin percentage estimates Oxygen carrying capacity in the blood of every patient. It is an indicator of total blood volume and amount of Oxygen available to the tissues.

In elective patients it is beneficial for reservation of blood and also in application of proper anaesthesia technique or precautions during monitoring of patient. Preoperative blood transfusion in indicated patients can be advised according to basic Haemoglobin percentage of patient. In chronically ill patients or patients with severe medical disorders of cardiovascular, respiratory, liver, kidney diseases or the patients posted for major operative procedures of thoracic, myocardial, neuro-surgery, orthopaedic, etc is very important for preoperative blood transfusion. It should be correlated with clinical findings.

Preoperative blood transfusion is very important in multiple trauma patients as part of preoperative preparation and resuscitation of patient.

2. Urine examination

Urine examination is done for presence of albumin, sugar and microscopic. When any abnormality is detected in routine urine examination, then these patients should be further investigated in detail. It is particularly important in liver, kidney, endocrine or electrolyte disturbances or patients on diuretic therapy.

In emergency patients, total urine output is important for evaluation of kidney functions which is beneficial in shock states, gastro-intestinal disorders, trauma states, etc. Urine should be seen for specific gravity, colour, odour. Reaction, Benedict's test, heat coagulation test, microscopic for casts, cells, ketone bodies, etc. On estimation of total important one can plan for technique of anaesthesia, drug administration, intravenous fluids, so that conduction of anaesthesia is smooth.

3. Blood Grouping and Typing

It should be carried out in every patient but it is more important in patients where blood transfusion may be required or where intra-operative or post-operative blood loss is anticipated or in patients with trauma or haemorhagic shock, concealed haemorhage, liver disease, anaemia, clotting abnormalities, major surgery, etc.

In preoperative states of anaemia or post-operative hypovolumia due to intra-operative blood loss, if blood grouping and Rh typing is already done then there should not be any delay in asking for blood transfusion. No one can be sure that there will not be bleeding even in minor procedures like cervical dilatation and curettage, lymph node biopsy or hernia repair, then preoperative blood grouping and typing will be beneficial to tackle emergency situation.

4. Blood Sugar (Random)

It is necessary to detect possibility of associated Diabetes mellitus in surgical patients particularly adult patients and geriatrics. When blood sugar value is more than expected then these patients should be investigated in detail for the status of disease and for control with appropriate therapy.

List of Investigations in Particular Systemic involvement

I. Cardiovascular System

- Haemoglobin percentage – for cardiopulmonary reserve and chronic illness
- Urine examination – Albumin estimation, when patient is in congestive cardiac failure and on diuretic therapy
- Blood grouping and typing
- ECG – For total estimation of myocardial status as arrhythmias, blocks, chamber hypertrophy, ischemia or infarction, conduction defects, etc.
- X-ray chest – For respiratory involvement secondary to cardiovascular disease, size of heart or chamber hypertrophy, calcification of valves, artifacts, thoracic cage, etc.

- Echocardiography
- Phonocardiography
- Heart scanning
- Cardiac catheterization for congenital abnormalities, pressure in various chambers, biopsy to detect various myopathies.
- Coronary angiography

II. Respiratory system

- Haemoglobin percentage – In chronic respiratory disease and detects cardiopulmonary reserve, it is of prognostic value in Pulmonary Tuberculosis
- Urine examination – Albumin estimation is related to patients with cardiac failure secondary to respiratory disorders and on diuretic therapy. Positive sugar in urine may be associated with diabetic patients are more prone for respiratory infections.
- Blood grouping and Rh typing
- Blood sugar – random
- X-ray chest – it is diagnostic of many of the respiratory diseases
- ECG – It is important in cardiac involvement secondary to respiratory pathology mainly obstructive airway disorders
- Pulmonary Function tests – as Tidal volume, PEFR and FEV_1 are important in diagnosis of either obstructive or restrictive airway disease. It is also of prognostic value. It is also important in evaluating postoperative pain relief in indicated and major surgery patients.
- Bronchoscopy
- Bronchography
- Ultra sonography
- Pleural Para centesis
- Match blowing test
- Breath holding time – important in evaluating cardiopulmonary reserve and preparation of patients for thoracic , pulmonary and major operations.

III. Liver Involvement

- Haemoglobin percentage – it is very important in liver diseases, haemolytic jaundice, cirrhosis of liver and other chronic liver disease
- Urine examination – urine albumin is important in cirrhosis of liver, hypoalbuminemia due to any cause.
- Bile salts and Bile pigments – in diagnosis of type of jaundice mainly obstructive
- Urine specific gravity – for diagnosis of jaundice
- Serum proteins – mainly serum albumin in chronic liver disease which is decreased, albumin/globulin ratio is reversed
- Serum cholesterol – important in patients with cholecystitis, gall stones
- Bleeding time
- Clotting time – In severe liver disease as cirrhosis of liver, malignancy, hepatitis, it is prolonged
- Prothrombine time is prolonged as this clotting factor production is decreased.
- Liver function tests – these are important in overall assessment of liver dysfunctions and are of prognostic value after starting of therapy.
  a. SGOT : indicates actual liver cell damage
  b. SGPT : indicates liver damage with obstructive pathology
  c. Serum alkaline phosphatase : indicates obstructive element
  d. LDH : indicates liver cell damage
  e. Serum bilirubin : indicates active or chronic liver cell damage and also alterations in bilirubin metabolism and bile excretion
- Blood urea – indicates associated kidney damage
- Blood urea nitrogen level – for kidney damage
- Serum electrolytes
- Serum creatinine – for estimation of kidney damage

- Liver ultra sonography
- Liver scanning and liver biopsy

IV. Kidney involvement

- 24 hours urine output important in shock states
- Urine examination for albumin, sugar, microscopic, physical characters, macroscopically (pH, specific gravity, colour, odour, reaction)
- Blood urea
- Serum creatinine
- Serum electrolytes – when patient is on diuretic therapy
- X-ray abdomen
- Pyelography – retrograde and intravenous antrograde
- Ultra sonography
- Kidney scanning

V. Diabetes mellitus

- Haemoglobin percentage for chronicity of disease and secondary infections
- Urine sugar estimation
- Blood sugar random
- Glucose tolerance test
- Urine for ketone bodies – Rothra's test
- Liver function tests for associated liver damage
- ECG
- Tests for Autonomic nervous system imbalance

VI. Thyroid Gland

- Thyroid function tests :
  a. Serum TSH
  b. Serum T_3
  c. Serum T_4
  d. Protein bound iodine

- ECG
- X-ray neck anterior and lateral view
- Indirect laryngoscopy
- Basal metabolic rate (BMR)
- Routine investigations

VII. Central nervous system

- Routine investigations
- Fundoscopy
- Tendon and other reflexes
- Sensory system
- Motor power
- Gait of the patient

After thorough examination and related investigations, patients are advised to take either, treatment for associated medical disorder so that patients are optimized for anaesthesia and surgery or these patients are accepted with due risk of associated medical disorder only during emergency situations. Many times the technique of anaesthesia or drug dosage is changed, due precautions during monitoring, so that morbidity and mortality related to anaesthesia and surgery is minimized.

Advice at the end of Preoperative assessment

1. All the patients posted for elective operative procedures are asked to be nil by mouth for at least 6 hours. This depends upon the age of the patient (paediatric, adult or geriatric), type of operative procedure whether elective or emergency. Usually patients with multiple trauma, pain in abdomen, fractures, patients in labour, paralytic ileus due to any cause, pyloric stenosis, hiatus hernia, intestinal obstruction, are considered to be with full stomach all the time.

   The emptying of stomach for various food ingredients is variable. For solid food material, the emptying time is 6–8 hours, for semi-solid (Biscuits, coffee, tea) it is up to 4 hours and for clear fluids within 1 hour. In paediatric patients, the emptying time of stomach is quicker and in geriatrics it is delayed as compared to adult patients.

Another aspect particularly during emergency is, whether pain, trauma, labour pains or stress, starts within emptying time of stomach, the these patients are considered to be with full stomach all the time, even kept nil by mouth.

Proper precautions to avoid vomiting and regurgitation should be taken in all these patients with full stomach so that dreadful complications as acid-aspiration syndrome Mandalson's syndrome) can be avoided.

2. **Consent of the patient :** Written and valid consent of the each patient for technique of anaesthesia and separate for operative procedure should be taken either posted during emergency or elective and minor or major procedures.

   Special precautions should be taken during consent of students staying at hostels, beggars, patients without relatives, accidents and paediatrics. Here valid consent from the guardian or parents, warden or Superintendent of hospital, competent persons should be obtained. This problem mainly arises during emergency situations.

   In the consent one should mention about the technique of anaesthesia to be employed in the patient with its advantages and complications, status of medical disorder, effects of drug therapy on technique of anaesthesia as well as drug interaction of these drugs with anaesthesia drugs, possible complications during intra-operatively and immediate postoperatively, available monitoring devices (particularly at small centers).

3. **Over night sedation :** It is advised mainly to anxious or in patients posted for major operative procedures. Minor tranquillizers or hypnotics are usually given. This will be beneficial to reduce the anxiety and will produce sound sleep on the night before operation. It is also beneficial to reduce the requirement of intravenous inducing agents and narcotic analgesics intra-operatively, which is useful particularly in patients with cardiovascular disorders. Sedatives and hypnotics

are relatively contraindicated in over night in patients with obstructive airway disease, other respiratory disorders, liver and kidney dysfunctions.

4. **Drug therapy :** Some these patients may be on various drug therapy for the treatment of associated medical disorders. In these situations, some drugs should be continued or omitted, on the day of operation to minimize drug interaction with the drugs used perioperatively for conduction of anaesthesia. Anti-arrhythmic, Anti-hypertensive, Anti-thyroid, Anti-anginal, Calcium channel blockers should be continued on the day of operation. Insulin, Digoxin, mycin group of antibiotics, Anti-convulsants, Sedatives, Hypnotics, Beta blockers, Anti-psychiatric drugs should be discontinued on the day of operation.

5. **Blood transfusion :** Preoperative blood transfusion should be advised 48 to 72 hours before the expected day of operation and anaesthesia so that it is most beneficial to the patient as far as physiological functions are concerned. This depends upon clinical pathology in the patient. In patients with acute blood loss, preoperative blood transfusion is not useful so adequate blood should be asked to reserve during intra-operative or immediate post-operative period.

In every patient, one should explain about the technique of anaesthesia (what technique you are adopting, how it is given, possible complications related to technique), its advantages, and complications to get maximum cooperation of the patient during its conduction. So it will minimize un-necessary medico-legal aspects during course of anaesthesia. Overall the technique of anaesthesia should be maximally beneficial to the patient with less chances of morbidity and mortality related to technique of anaesthesia.

5

Intravenous Inducing Agents

In general intravenous anaesthetic agents are used for the induction of general anaesthesia, as sole anaesthetic agent (total intravenous anaesthesia), to supplement volatile anaesthesia or regional anaesthesia and for sedation. Many of the agents have been used intravenously to produce unconsciousness and a safe reversible anaesthetic state. Six commands are commonly used –

- Aliphatic substances : Alcohol, Chloral hydrate
- Barbiturates
- Opiates
- Steroids
- Aromatic compounds
- Neuroleptic drugs

THIOPENTONE SODIUM

It is sodium ethyl thiobarbiturate. It is sulphur analogue of pentobarbitone introduced by Dundee in 1935.

Physical Properties

- It is yellow amorphous powder with odour of H_2S.
- It is soluble in water and alcohol, 2.5% - 5% solution with pH 10.5 which is highly alkaline.

- It is prepared in 6% anhydrous sodium carbonate in Nitrogen atmosphere, to prevent formation of free acid by carbon dioxide of atmosphere.
- In solution it is not very stable but can be kept for 24–48 hrs without any change in potency when solution is clear.
- When the solution is cloudy then it should be discarded.
- Oil/water coefficient is 4.7
- It is supplied in ampoules with distilled water
- Average Dose is 5–7 mg / kg intravenously.

Pharmacological actions

Central Nervous System

- It causes sedation, hypnosis, anaesthesia, respiratory depression depending upon the dose and rate of injection.
- It has anti-convulsant action.
- Cerebral cortex and ascending reticular activating system are depressed before medullary center.
- Cerebral blood flow and cerebral spinal fluid pressure are reduced.
- It has anta – analgesic property.
- It causes dose dependent depression of EEG waves.
- Acute tolerance – with larger induction dose, the patient awakes at a higher blood levels. A high initial concentration and Thiopentone in brain may result in an increased acute tolerance to supplement doses.
- Metabolic actions reduces Thiopentone concentration in plasma by 40%.
- About 87% of drug in peripheral blood is bound to plasma proteins, mainly albumin and so is inactivated, pH changes may affect the ratio of bound to unbound Thiopentone, maximum with pH 8. The degree of binding also varies according to the concentration of Thiopentone being greatest when concentration is low.

- It causes dose and concentration dependent depression of respiratory center which is antagonized by surgical stimuli and potentiated by opioids.

Respiratory System

- It has no direct effect on respiratory system. Initially there is stimulation of respiration first, tachypnoea, CO_2 wash out, apnoea, CO_2 accumulation and then regular respiration.
- It may cause laryngospasm in irritable respiratory tract or bronchospasm secondary to histamine release or in patient with bronchial asthma.

Cardiovascular System

- It reduces myocardial contractility, which is compensated by tachycardia and increases the myocardial oxygen consumption.
- Peripheral vascular resistance is slightly reduced leading to pooling of blood in periphery, reduction in cardiac out put particularly in hypovolumia and in patients with hypotension due to any cause.
- It is dangerous in patient when heart can not compensate for changes in vascular haemodynamics i.e. patients on beta blockers, constrictive pericarditis, tight valvular disease, complete heart block, hypotension depending upon dose and concentration of drug injected.
- It may cause direct vaso-motor center depression.
- There is more decrease in blood pressure in patients with un-controlled hypertension and untreated hypertension.
- On rapid induction and intubation, it may cause laryngospasm in sensitive patients.
- Pupils first dilate and then constrict after Thiopentone. It reduces intra-occular tension, loss of eyelash reflex, a sign of induction of anaesthesia.
- Thiopentone has no effect on tone of pregnant uterus. It readily

crosses placental barrier, achieving its maximum concentration in foetal blood very soon after injection.

- It has no direct effect on liver and kidney functions. It is powerful stimulator of ADH.

Metabolism, fate and Excretion

- After a single small dose, its level in the plasma falls rapidly and the patients regain consciousness, as a result of redistribution to viscera, muscles and fat during first 10 minutes after injection.
- After a single dose or repeated small doses, plasma blood levels may be high enough to cause prolonged anaesthesia.
- It rapidly crosses blood brain barrier due to its low degree of ionization and high lipid solubility. Equilibrium between plasma and brain is established 1 minute after intravenous injection. The initial high uptake of Thiopentone by brain is due to high lipid solubility and non-ionization and responsible for rapid onset of anaesthesia.
- The metabolism starts after 15 minutes in the liver. 10–15% of drug is metabolized in each hour. The products of metabolism are excreted by kidney. It passes into breast milk after injection.
- It has drug interaction with Barbiturates and Warfarin and there is potentiation of action. There is minimum histamine release. Hypersensitivity reactions are less.

Indications

- For induction of anaesthesia.
- For induction in balanced technique of anaesthesia.
- As a sole anaesthetic agent in short surgical procedures as incision and drainage of abscess, reduction of fractures, urethral dilatation, cervical dilatation, joint dislocations, etc.
- As anti-convulsant in acute convulsions due to hypoxia, tetanus, eclampsia, epilepsy or in drip form in continuous convulsions in status epileptics, tetanus and eclampticus.

- For electro-convulsive therapy.
- Brain resuscitation due to its scavenging action.
- For Psychoanalysis.
- As a supplement to regional anaesthesia.
- Day care surgery as induction agent.

Contraindications

- Absolute :
  - Acute intermittent Porphyria, it may induce crisis. It may precipitate lower motor neuron paralysis and death.
  - Thiopentone anaphylaxis known case.
  - Access of veins is difficult
- Relative :
  - Shock, debilitated, severe anaemia, mal-nourishement patients.
  - Severe hypotension or shock due to hypovolumia, cardiogenic, anaphylactic or neurogenic.
  - Extremes of age – as venous access is difficult
  - Respiratory crippled patients as in severe obstructive or restrictive airway diseases , acute bronchial asthma, lobectomy, pneumonectomy etc
  - Low fixed cardiac out put states as Mitral stenosis, Aortic stenosis, constrictive pericarditis, pericardial effusion, cardiac tamponade, etc.
  - In patients with heart disease as complete heart block, myocardial ischemia and infarction, severe hypertension, myocarditis, congestive cardiac failure due to any cause, left ventricular failure, etc.
- Acute intestinal obstruction, chances of regurgitation.
- Upper respiratory tract infection.
- External podalic version, manual removal of placenta.
- Dystrophia myotonica
- Severe alcoholics
- Anticipated difficult intubation

- Metabolic and electrolyte disturbances
- When resuscitation facilities are not available
- Hypokalamic familial periodic paralysis
- Severe hepatic and renal disease
- Huntington's chorea
- Thermal injury and burns

Advantages

- It gives smooth and rapid induction of anaesthesia
- There is absence of delirium phase
- It produces rapid recovery from anaesthesia.
- The depth of anaesthesia can be increased or decreased by control rate of administration of drug.

Disadvantages

- It may produce severe respiratory depression
- Some times there may be laryngospasm
- Circulatory and myocardial depression.

Complications

- Local complications – It may cause pain, redness, haematoma formation, bruising and then ulceration if injected intra-dermally and when there is extravasation.
- Median nerve injury, when given at anti-cubital fossa
- Accidental intra-arterial injection, it is common at anti-cubital fossa or in the presence of arterio-venous fistula. There is severe burning sensation and pain along the course of artery, arteriolar spasm secondary to high alkalinity of solution, arterial thrombosis and occlusion due to precipitate obstruction and release of cathecholamines.

  It is treated as –

    Keep the needle as it in the vein or artery

- Intravenous Heparin 500 I.U.
- Dilution with normal saline infusion
- Papeverin 40–80 mg in 10–20 ml of normal saline
- Tolazoline or Priscol 5 ml in 1% solution
- Phenoxy benzamine 0.5 mg or drip of 50–200 μgm/min
- Brachial plexus block for relief of pain
- Thrombophlebitis – may occur when given in small veins in higher concentration
- General complications
- Respiratory depression – dose and concentration dependent, central medullary depression
- Depression of vasomotor center
- Laryngospasm in irritable respiratory tract
- Bronchospasm in bronchial asthma patients
- Postoperative vertigo, euphoria and dis-orientation
- Hyper-sensitivity or anaphylactic reactions
- Severe myocardial or peripheral circulatory depression or collapse.

PROPANIDID

It is non-barbiturate, ultra-short acting intravenous anaesthetic agent and derived from Eugonal. Chemically it is propyl–4–diethyl carbamoyl methoxy–3–methoxy phenyl acetate. It is yellowish oil in 20% cremophor EL solution of ethosylated castor oil. Molecular weight is 337.4, Boiling point 210^0 c and pH is 7.8.

- Dose is 5–7 mg/kg, it can be diluted in distilled water or normal saline.
- When it is administered intravenously, it causes initial hyperventilation followed by hypoventilation or apnoea. There is slight increase in pulse rate and blood pressure. It rapidly produces unconsciousness of short duration. There is no hang over effect. The rapid recovery is due to rapid distribution to

all well perfused organs and detoxificated by cholinesterase in liver. The metabolites has no anaesthetic property. The break down products are excreted via kidneys.

- It does not give excessive salivation and upper respiratory secretions. There is no postoperative vomiting.
- It may give abnormal limb movements.
- It is not anta-analgesic.
- It prolongs the duration of action of Suxamethonium secondary to same pathway of destruction by plasma cholinesterase.
- It may cause irritation along with the course of vein or phlebitis due to high viscosity.
- It is mainly discarded from anaesthesia practice due to high incidence of hyper-sensitivity reactions. These reactions are attributed to stabilizing agent Cremophor EL.
- It is commonly used as inducing agent for short surgical procedures and electro-convulsive therapy.
- Now a days this drug is not available.

ALTHESIN

- It is potent steroid intravenous anaesthetic agent. It is mixture of alphaxalone and alphadolone in Cremophor EL.
- Dose is 0.05–0.075 ml / kg very slowly.
- It immediately produces smooth induction of anaesthesia.
- It is short acting and the effect lasts for 7–12 minutes.
- It does not cause pain along the course of injection so there are less chances of postoperative phlebitis.
- There is fall in blood pressure, central venous pressure and compensatory increase in pulse rate.
- The hyper-sensitivity reactions as severe anaphylactic shock is secondary to preservative Cremophor EL.
- The drug itself has no specific actions on respiratory and cardiovascular functions
- 1 ml contains 9 mg of alphaoxalone and 3 mg alphaldolone. The anaesthetic properties are with alphaoxalone. Recovery

is fast as there is no redistribution. 20 to 30% of metabolism takes place in liver, excretion via kidney. 60 to 70% of drug is excreted via bile and feces over days together. Recovery from anaesthesia is completed within 10 minutes.

- It is mainly used as sedation in ICU, total intravenous anaesthesia as hypnotic.
- It is suitable for Day care surgery.
- Postoperative nausea and vomiting is rare.
- Now a days it is not available and not commonly used due to its high incidence of hypersensitivity reactions.

ETOMIDATE

It is carboxylated imidazole. 10 ml ampoule contains 2 mg / kg dissolved in water with 35% propylene glycol. PH is 8.1. It is non-barbiturate intravenous anaesthetic agent.

- It is said to be safer than Althesin and other drugs.
- It is potent and rapidly acting intravenous hypnotic drug. The elimination half life is 2 to 5 hours and 96% is bound to plasma proteins.
- The onset of action is within one arm-brain circulation time.
- Dose is 0.2–0.4 mg/kg and the duration of action lasts for 7–12 minutes.
- It does not cause either respiratory or cardiovascular depression but larger doses may cause apnoea and tachycardia.
- It is haemodynamically stable and maintains heart rate, blood pressure, stroke volume and cardiac output. Some times there is 10–15%decrease is systolic blood pressure due to decrease in peripheral vascular resistance.
- There is no analgesic action.
- It does not affect normal liver and kidney functions.
- There is no histamine release but reduction in cortisol production is noted.
- It is redistributed in the body and metabolized in liver. The metabolites are biologically inactive and excreted via kidneys.

Disadvantages

- It causes pain at the site of injection, myoclonic movements, cough, hic-coughs or strider. These side effects can be prevented by premedication with Diazepam. Postoperative nausea and vomiting is common.
- The drug is no more used in anaesthesia practice due to non-availability.

DIAZEPAM

- It is benzodiazepene derivative. Now a days used as intravenous inducing agent in some group of patients.
- It is insoluble in water and so it is prepared in organic solvent or emulsifying agent. Organic solvents are irritant on intravenous injection and causes thrombophlebitis.
- Induction dose is 0.3–0.5 mg / kg, elimination half life is 21 to 37 hours, clearance is 0.2–0.5 ml/kg/minute and volume of distribution is 1–1.5 ml / kg

Pharmacological actions

1. Central nervous system

The central actions are mediated by facilitation of the inhibition of synaptic transmission by Gamma amino butyric acid (GABA). It relives tension and anxiety and causes drowsiness with control of convulsions. It is nor analgesic. It potentiates the actions of other sedatives, hypnotics and anaesthetic agents. It depresses the limbic system and amygdala to relive fear, anxiety and aggression. There is no cortical depression. It produces anterograde amnesia. There is no nausea and vomiting. It does not increases the cerebral blood flow but intra-cranial pressure is decreased due to decrease in systemic blood pressure.

2. Respiratory System

It causes dose dependent respiratory center depression. It produces some broncho-dilatation, the rate and depth of respiration is decreased. It produces skeletal muscle relaxation so there is decrease in tidal volume and minute ventilation. In therapeutic doses there is no change in respiratory functions.

3. *Cardiovascular System*

- It causes dose dependent vasomotor center depression, direct myocardial depression, peripheral vasodilatation, decrease in cardiac output in very high doses. In therapeutic doses, it has efficient cardiovascular stability, so a drug of choice as premedication. So it is used as inducing agent in open-heart surgery.
- It has anti-hypertensive and anti-arrhythmic property, mainly anxiety oriented.
- Neuro-muscular junction – It potentiates the actions of non-depolarizing and reduces the incidence of fasciculations after Suxamethonium. It relieves muscle spasm and spasticity.
- It crosses the placental barrier and may produce muscle relaxation in new born and occasionally floppy baby syndrome. So it is avoided up to delivery of foetus during caesarian section.
- It is metabolized in liver and excreted in bile. The main metabolite N – desmethyl – diazepam is excreted in urine. 98% of drug is bound to plasma proteins and rapid distribution in fat.

Clinical Uses

- 'Dose is 0.1–0.3 mg/kg oral or parental.
- It is mainly used as premedication, before induction of anaesthesia.
- As an adjuvant to regional anaesthesia.
- Cardioversion
  - As sedative for endoscopies.
  - To control postoperative restlessness.
  - As anti-convulsant in status tetanus, status eclampticus, status epilepticus

- Cardiac catheterization
  - To treat and reduce hallucinations after Ketamine anaesthesia
  - For short surgical procedures as induction agent in shoulder dislocation, manual removal of placenta, etc.
  - Open heart surgery – mitral valvotomy as inducing agent.
  - In treatment of hypertension, ventricular tachy-arrhythmias, anxiety states, pre-eclamptic toxaemia, etc.
- Side effects : It may produce profound drowsiness, muscle weakness, headache, vertigo, nausea and vomiting, when give in very high doses.

KETAMINE HYDROCHLORIDE

It is non–barbiturate intravenous inducing agent. It is water soluble, pH 3.5 to 5.5 and stored at room temperature and protected from light and heat. It is phencyclidine derivative and produces dissociative type of anaesthesia.

Pharmacological actions

1. Central nervous system

It causes depression of thalamo-cortical system, mainly motor and sensory cortex and activates part of limbic system. Thus it produces functional dissociation. Dissociative anaesthesia is a cataleptic state with profound analgesia. The patient may appear awake, eyes often remain open, nystagmus, unpurposeful muscle movements. The elimination half life is 1–2 hours. It produces unconsciousness and total analgesia.

2. Respiratory system

In usual doses, the respiration is stimulated but may be depressed in neonates and in very high doses. It increases the lung compliance and decreases the airway resistance. There is Preservation of upper airway reflexes.

3. Cardiovascular system

- It increases the blood pressure due to central sympathetic stimulation and depression of baro-receptors. There is increase in pulse rate, It increases the cardiac out put due to increase in pulse rate. There is no change in peripheral vascular resistance. It may sensitize the myocardium to exogenous catecholamines. It has no vagolytic action.
- It increases intra-occular pressure.
- It increases the cerebral blood flow and there by increase in intra-cranial pressure.
- There may be spontaneous muscular movements like tremors or twitching. There is muscular relaxation, in spite there is some rigidity.
- There is stimulation of Edinger-Westpal nucleus, so postoperative nausea and vomiting is common. There is increase in salivary secretions so atropinization is to be given as premedication.
- It is usually given in 1% solution, in dose of 2 mg / kg and the onset of action starts within 30 seconds. It can be given orally or intra-muscularly in doses of 10 mg / kg and 5 mg / kg respectively. Here the onset of action is within 3 minutes and the duration of action is for about 30 minutes. It can be given is drip form as 50 ¼gm / kg / minute for analgesia in balanced technique of anaesthesia.
- It is metabolized in liver and excreted via kidneys. It is converted into water soluble nor-Ketamine by N-demethylation and hydroxylation and excreted in urine.

Clinical Uses

- As a sole anaesthetic agent for short surgical procedures.
- As a induction agent in general anaesthesia.
- In anticipated difficult endotracheal intubation.
- Neurological radio-diagnostic procedures.
- In critically ill patients, debilitated and patients with any type of shock.

- In open heart surgery.
- For orthopaedic manipulations, fracture reduction or joint dislocations
- During multiple anaesthetic exposures like burn dressings, cleaning and debridement and cleaning of wounds.
- Mass casualties.
- As only analgesic in balanced technique of anaesthesia or as a supplementation for regional anaesthesia.
- In drip form for postoperative pain relief or epidurally.
- For total intravenous anaesthesia in Day care surgery.
- Bier's block – intravenous regional anaesthesia.
- Oral Ketamine as premedication in paediatric patients.

Contraindications

- In patients with psychological disturbances.
- In major surgical procedures.
- Thyrotoxicosis and thyroid dysfunctions
- In patients with severe cardiovascular disorders as acute myocardial infarction, hypertension, arrhythmias, etc.
- In patients with raised intra-cranial pressure due to any cause.
- Neuromuscular disorders or dystrophy.

Advantages

- It can be used as sole anaesthetic agent in difficult environment with minimum monitoring devices.
- Induction of anaesthesia is pleasant with cardiovascular stability.
- There is alterations in the respiratory parameters.
- It has high therapeutic index and suitable in poor risk patients.
- It can be given for repeated administrations.
- It cane be preoperatively, intraoperatively and postoperatively for pain relief.

Disadvantages

- Emergence delirium
- Hallucinations – aural or visual
- Increase in blood pressure, intra-cranial pressure and intra-occular pressure
- Hypertonia of muscles
- Respiratory depression in neonates
- Nausea and vomiting
- Increase in tone of uterine contractions
- It increases sympathetic activity so exogenous adrenaline is contraindicated along with Ketamine anaesthesia.

MIDAZOLAM

- It is new water soluble benzodiazepene compound which can be used for induction of anaesthesia and as sedation during premedication. The solubility is pH dependent, below 4 it is freely soluble but at body pH it is lipid soluble and rapidly penetrates blood brain barrier.
- It is 2–3 times more potent than Diazepam. It incorporates an imidazole ring which confirms the solubility in aqueous solutions.
- It is not irritant on intravenous injection like Diazepam and does not contain any stabilizing agent.
- It is well absorbed after intravenous administration.
- 95% of it is bound to plasma proteins and metabolized in liver by hepatic P_{450}.
- Onset of action is within 1–2 minutes and duration of action is for 1–2 hours. Sedation dose is 0.05–0.1 mg/kg, induction dose is 0.15–0.3 mg /kg and infusion dose is 2–5¼ gm/kg. The onset of sleep is slow and there is a wide variation in response with sleep (80 secs to 3 mints). Recovery is faster than Diazepam.
- It causes sedation, anxiolysis and anaesthesia depending upon the dose.

- It has no analgesic action.
- Recovery is usually within 6–8 minutes after intravenous induction.
- Anterograde amnesia and drowsiness is common.
- It. has cardiovascular stability. It causes slight decrease is systemic vascular resistance and fall in arterial blood pressure. There is no change in cardiac out put.
- There is no marked respiratory depression and it is similar to equipotent doses of Diazepam. The elderly patients are more prone for respiratory depression. So it should be give carefully in patients with chronic obstructive airway diseases.
- It has anti-convulsant and anti-hallucination property.
- It decreases cerebral blood flow and cerebral metabolism.
- It can be given orally and is well absorbed. It can be used intra-nasally or rectally.

Clinical uses

- It is widely used for premedication before induction of anaesthesia.
- It is used for sedation during endoscopies, laproscopy, bronchoscopy and procedures under general anaesthesia.
- For induction of anaesthesia in short surgical procedures in day care surgery.
- For conscious sedation.
- It can be used as anti-convulsant as it is potent.

PROPOFOL

It is a hindered phenol, insoluble in water. It is present as aqueous emulsion containing 10% soyabean oil, 1.2% egg phosphatide and 2.25% glycerol. It is potent anaesthetic agent like Thiopentone sodium.

- It is 98% protein bound and weak acid pKa 11.
- It produces smooth and rapid induction of anaesthesia within one arm-brain circulation time. Induction is within 30 seconds

after 2–2.5 mg / kg intravenously followed by recovery within 4–8 minutes.

- It produces pain along the course of vein of injection and so less pain is perceived if prior Lignocaine is administered in same vein.
- It reduces cerebral blood flow and cerebral spinal fluid pressure. It decreases oxygen consumption by reducing cerebral metabolic rate. It may produce excitation due to glycine antagonism at subcortical sites.
- It depresses the respiration by direct action on the medullary respiratory center and production of apnoea may be there. It decreases the sensitivity of respiratory center to effects of carbon dioxide.
- It does not later normal liver functions.
- There are less chances of postoperative nausea and vomiting.
- There is no effect on resting broncho-motor tone but depresses the laryngeal reflexes..
- It significantly decreases the systemic blood pressure due to fall in systemic vascular resistance. There is reduction in cardiac out put with tachy-arrhythmic response. It decreases myocardial oxygen demand, myocardial blood flow and coronary vascular resistance. Thus it is potent cardiovascular depressant and so used very cautiously in patients with cardiovascular disorders.
- There is no effect on gravid uterus contraction but rapidly crosses placental barrier.
- Liver and kidney functions are affected after its use.
- Recovery from anaesthesia is rapid and pleasant.
- After intravenous administration, it is rapidly distributed from blood to tissues and metabolized in liver and metabolites are excreted in urine.

Clinical Uses

- For intravenous induction of anaesthesia.

- For induction and maintinance of anesthesia in Day care surgery. The hypnotic property is useful in total intravenous anaesthesia.
- It can be given in infusion for minor surgical procedures.
- As sedative in regional anaesthesia
- For control of convulsions
- For sedation in critically ill patients, in shock states, ICU, radio-diagnostic procedures, endoscopies, etc.

Contraindications

- Unless and until indicated it should not be given.
- When resuscitation facilities are not available.
- Patients with severe cardiovascular disorders
- Known case with allergic manifestations
- Along with other histamine releasing drugs
- In elderly patients.

Side effects

- Nausea and vomiting is common or may be secondary to cardiovascular effects
- There are chances of thrombophlebitis
- There are chances of histamine release and anaphylactic reactions
- Minor or significant muscle movements from twitching to convulsions
- Central anti-cholinergic response
- Severe myocardial depression, bradycardia, hypotension, reduction in systemic vascular resistance, reduction in release of circulating catecholamines, arrhythmias and there are chances of hypertensive obstructive cardio-myopathy.
- Usual anaesthetic effects will not be encountered even though adequate doses of drugs are given.
- Emergence from anaesthesia is more rapid than Thiopentone so it is ultra short acting.

NEUROLEPT ANAESTHESIA

In 1949, Laborit put a concept that general anaesthesia can protect one from surgical pain by depression of cortical or sub-cortical centers alone.

Neurolepsis is defined as the suppression of sub-cortical and central autonomic activity with minimum toxic effects, when potent tranquillizer is combined with potent narcotic analgesic – a state of neurolept analgesia is produced – patient lies at rest and is completely passive.

Characteristics of Neurolept analgesia

- Psychic indifference to environmental stimuli
- Marked tranquility without loss of consciousness (apparent somnolence)
- Psychomotor placidity or hypokinesis – motor sedation is referred to as mineralozation.
- Suppressed reflexes
- Homeostasis – cardiovascular stability
- Amnesia
- Analgesia
- Basal anaesthesia
- Initially combination of Haloperidol as neuroleptic and Phenoperidine as narcotic was used but there were marked circulatory depression, extra-pyramidal symptoms and postoperative psychic changes.
- Now a day Droperidol (2.5 mg) and Fentanyl (0.5 mg) is the best combination in use.
- Recommended Technique of Administration
- Appropriate premedication
- Separate administration of drugs
- Neurolepsis with Droperidol (with slow onset of action and prolonged duration of action) and analgesia with Fentanyl (with short duration of action)

- Maintenance with Fentanyl alone
- Supplementation with Oxygen/Nitrous oxide
- Endotracheal intubation with topical anaesthesia
- Assisted or controlled ventilation

Advantages

- The technique is safe, simple, non-explosive and economical
- Prolonged major surgical procedures can be carried out with minimum risk of toxicity
- Prolonged analgesia with out cardiovascular impairment and cortical depression
- Pain relief can be extended in the postoperative period
- The adrenergic blocking action of Droperidol gives cardiovascular stability. It has peripheral tissue relaxation effect which provides optimal tissue perfusion.
- Droperidol also has anti-arrhythmic property which is beneficial in cardiac surgery.
- The patient can be awakened during surgery
- There are less chances of nausea and vomiting in total perioperative period
- There is total amnesia for induction and recovery phase of anaesthesia
- Fentanyl induced respiratory depression is rare and antagonized easily by narcotic antagonists.

Disadvantages

- Profound respiratory depression which may require Ventilatory support in the susceptible patients
- Pulmonary compliance may be decreased during phase of respiratory depression
- In poor risk patients, there may be severe circulatory collapse with low doses
- It does not provide any muscle relaxation

Complications

- Fentanyl induced respiratory depression may lead to severe hypoxia
- Inability to ventilate the lungs during respiratory depression phase due to rigidity of chest musculature and ventilation muscle relaxants have to be used
- When other narcotics are used along with it, may cause severe respiratory depression requiring intensive management
- In poor risk patients and in elderly, there are chances of cardiovascular collapse
- Extra-pyramidal muscular movements may develop during induction and maintenance of anaesthesia
- Some times blurring of vision, muscular hyper activity, diaphoresis, emergence delirium may be rarely noted.

6

Local Anaesthetic Agents

These are chemical agents capable of blocking nerve conduction, when applied locally to nerve tissue in a concentration that will not potentially damage the nerve tissue. Cocaine was the first drug naturally occurring having this property.

These drugs block the pain sensation along with touch, pressure and temperature sensation. In 1884, Koller applied Cocaine to the conjunctiva and produced local anaesthesia. The desirable characteristics of local anaesthetic are –

- Potent, effective in low concentration
- Good permeability
- Rapid onset of action
- Satisfactorily prolonged duration of action
- Low systemic toxicity or side effects
- Non-irritating or nerve damage
- Easily sterilized
    - These drugs are lipid soluble bases and act by penetrating the lipoprotein cell membranes excitable tissues in non-ionized state. These depress the transmission of nerve impulses in both sensory and motor nerves by preventing the migration of Sodium ions across the nerve membrane and also act by competing with Calcium ions.
    - The fine fibers are blocked first than thicker fibers.

· Local anaesthetics diffuse through the cell wall of neuron and inside the axon, the drug molecules are protonated, enter the Sodium channel and bind to trans-membrane pore. These bind with Sodium channel only when it is open or inactive. When the channel contains local anaesthetic drug, it becomes closed and conduction is inhibited. Rapid repetitive stimulation has more access for local anaesthetic and enhances the neural block.

· Quantitative and Qualitative differences chemically and variations in tolerance, potency and toxicity provide a wide spectrum of local anaesthetic available.

These are divided in 3 groups –

I) Esters :
- Benzoic acid esters :
  a – Soluble type : Procaine, Chlorprocaine
  b – Limited soluble : Benzocaine
- Para ethoxy benzoic acid : Intracaine
- Carbonic acid esters : Diathonae
- Complex synthetics

II) Amides :
- Straight chain acid derivatives of Xylidide
  a – Acetic acid : Xylocaine, Lignocaine or Lidocaine
  b – Propionic acid : Propitocaine
- Pipe colic acid derivative of Xylidide : Mepivacaine, Bupivacaine
- Oxy cinchonionic acid : Dibucaine

III) Alcohols – Ethyl alcohol, aromatic alcohol – benzyl alcohol

IV) Miscellaneous –
- Complex synthetics : Holocaine
- Quinoline derivative : Eucupin

LIGNOCAINE HYDROCHLORIDE–XYLOCAINE

• It is synthetic local anaesthetic agent prepared in 1943 by Lofgren and first used by Gordh in 1948.

- It is Diethyl amino–2–6–aceto xylidide. It is in amide group local anaesthetic agent.
- It is effective even on topical application
- It has no effect on blood vessels
- There is amnesia and drowsiness due to cerebral depression. It may produce general analgesia when given intravenously.
- When applied topically on cornea, it causes midriasis, vaso-constriction and cycloplegia.
- It is freely soluble in water and pH is 6.5–7.0
- It is stable on autoclaving or boiling. It is non-irritant to nerve tissue. The systemic toxicity is 1/5 that of Cocaine and 1.5 times of Procaine. It is 3 times more potent than Procaine.
- Total dose ranges from 500–750 mg in adult, maximum safe dose is 7 mg/kg with Adrenaline and 3–5 mg/kg without Adrenaline. Here Adrenaline is used to delay vascular absorption and to prolong the duration of action. The onset of action is rapid and duration lasts for 60–120 minutes.
- It is metabolized in liver and excreted via kidney. About 5% of drug is excreted unchanged in urine. Most of the drug is metabolized by transformation into free and conjugated phenol and ring is hydroxylated.

Pharmacological actions

Central nervous system

Central nervous system is stimulated producing restlessness, tremors and in toxic doses convulsions. Central stimulation is followed by depression.

Cardiovascular system

- These are direct myocardial depressant agents. Heart rate and amplitude of contractions is decreased, the excitability threshold and refractory period are prolonged and conduction is slowed.
- Larger doses produce changes in ECG and some times

precipitate ventricular fibrillation and cardiac standstill in diastole in very toxic doses but in therapeutic doses it is the drug choice for treatment of ventricular tachycardia or extra systoles. It provides anti-arrhythmic action.

- It causes extrusion of calcium from sarcoplasmic reticulum.
- It has some anti-bacterial action. It is said that, it inhibits phagocytosis and metabolism of leukocytes.

Recommended concentrations

- Infiltration : 0.5%
- Nerve block : 1–1.5%
- Spinal block : 5%
- Epidural or Caudal block : 1.5–2%
- Cornea : 2–4%
- Insufflations or spray : 4%
- Mucosa : 2% jelly
- Intravenous regional : 0.5% total dose 3 mg / kg, 25–40 ml for upper limb and 50 60 ml for lower limb.
- Continuous infusion or drip : 1 mg/kg/hr.

Clinical uses

- Regional anaesthesia as Spinal, epidural, nerve block, infiltration, mucosal, surface anaesthesia, etc.
- For laryngoscopy or bronchoscopy under local anaesthesia
- For short surgical procedures – anal dilatation, cervical dilatation, urethral dilatation in jelly form
- For ophthalmic procedures
- For short surgical procedures performed under local anaesthesia as suturing, biopsy, corn removal, etc.
- Intravenous regional anaesthesia in orthopaedic surgery, general surgery confined to extremities
- As an analgesic in balanced technique of anaesthesia

- For obstetric analgesia
- In the treatment of various arrhythmias as ventricular extra systoles, ventricular tachycardia or fibrillation.
- In cardiac resuscitation
- To attenuate pressor response to laryngoscopy and endotracheal intubation in patients with hypertension, ischemic heart disease or tachycardia due to any cause.
- As anti-convulsant in drip form in eclampsia, tetanus or epilepsy
- To decrease fasciculations after Suxamethonium
- To decrease rise in intra-gastric pressure, intra-occular pressure and muscle pain after Suxamethonium.

Adverse effects

- In therapeutic doses it is very safe drug. There are less chances of adverse effects or anaphylactic reactions with it. The preservatives along with drug are many times responsible for adverse effects as anaphylactic reactions.
- In very high doses, it may cause firstly stimulation of central nervous system followed by depression.
- It may produce some sedation.
- As such there are no contraindications to it.

BUPIVACAINE

It is new synthetic local anaesthetic introduced by Ekenstan in 1957 and used by Telivio in 1963. It is very stable even to repeated autoclaving, in acids and alkalis.

- It is four times more potent than Lignocaine and Mepivacaine. It has increased lipid solubility and protein binding as compared to Lignocaine so there is prolonged duration of action.
- The onset of action is within 3–5 minutes and duration of action from 3–5 hours. It has no effect of addition of adrenaline.
- Dose is 2 mg / kg of body weight by any route.
- It is given in concentrations of 0.5%, 0.75% and 0.25%.

- It is anilide compound and chemical name is 1–n–butyl–DL–piperdone–2–carbolic acid–2–6 dimethyl anilide hydrochloride. Molecular weight is 325 and melting point is 258°C and pH 3.5.
- It is reliable drug for infiltration and nerve blocks but unpredictable for spinal anaesthesia. It has slow nerve penetrating power. Excellent sensory block is produced with poor muscle relaxation. Even in concentration of 0.25%, it produces good sensory block and for muscle relaxation more than 0.5% concentration is required.
- It is metabolized in liver. On continuous drip administration, it is cleared from plasma. Most of the drug is metabolized by N–dealkylation.
- It crosses placental barrier as passive diffusion but there are no effects on foetus. About 10% of drug is excreted unchanged in urine within 24 hours.
- Recommended concentrations :
  Infiltration : 0.25%
  Nerve blocks : 0.25–0.5%
  Spinal block : 0.5%
  Epidural and caudal : 0.25–0.5%

Clinical uses

- Now a days, hyperbaric 0.5% solution is used for spinal anaesthesia and plane 0.5% solution is used for epidural and nerve blocks.
- Intravenous regional anaesthesia
- Obstetric analgesia.

Contraindications

It is relatively contraindicated in patients with cardiovascular disorders, anaemia with hypo-proteinaemia due to any cause and in liver diseases.

Adverse reactions

- It is irritable directly to myocardium and causes stimulation of cardiovascular system. It causes severe bradycardia and hypotension due to direct action on myocardium. This action is noted with concentrations more than 0.75%.
- It has some cumulative effect in higher concentrations
- It affects sympathetic nervous system.
- Shivering may be secondary to hypotension and peripheral vasodilatation.
- The older local anaesthetics which were previously used but due to toxicity are not in current use are, Cocaine, Procaine, Chlorprocaine, Amethocaine, Cinchocaine, Prilocaine, Tetracaine, Nupercaine or Dibucaine, etc.
- Now days newer local anaesthetic agents are under trial and these are Levobupivacaine, Mepivacaine and Ropivacaine.
- Most commonly used local anaesthetic agents are Lignocaine and Bupivacaine as there is no other choice of local anaesthetics in India in present situations.

7

Subarchanoid or Spinal and Epidural Block

D. Cotuguo discovered cerebro-spinal fluid in 1764 and F. Magendie in 1825 described the circulation and who also gave the name. T.L. Corning, neurologist in 1885, gave first successful spinal block. First planed spinal anaesthesia for surgery was performed by August Bier on 16th August 1898.

Anatomy

- The vertebral column consists of 7 cervical, 12 thoracic, 5 lumbar, 5 sacral and 4 or 5 coccygeal vertebrae.
- Vertebral column has four curves, thoracic and sacral curves are primary curves and are concave anteriorly. When spine is fully flexed, the cervical and lumbar curves are obliterated.
- In supine position, 3rd lumbar vertebra marks the highest point of lumbar curve, 5th thoracic is the lowest point of dorsal curve.
- Kyphosis, lardosis, scoliosis and hypertrophic arthritis changes normal curvature of these curves and makes lumbar puncture difficult to perform.
- The spinous processes of cervical, upper 2 thoracic and last four vertebrae are horizontal. The other spinous processes are inclined downwards. The tips are opposite to next lower vertebral body.

Important Surface markings

- C_7 : Vertebral prominence
- T_3 : Tip of spine is opposite to spine of scapula with arms by the side of body
- T_7 : Inferior angle of scapula with arms to side
- L_4 or L_4–L_5 : Highest point of iliac crest
- Dimple over lying posterior superior iliac spine is on line crossing the second posterior sacral foramina.

Vertebral canal

It is bounded in front by bodies of vertebrae and inter-vertebral discs, posteriorly by the laminae, ligamentum flavum and arch which bears the spinous processes, inter-spinous ligaments, laterally by pedicles and laminae.

The contents of vertebral canal are – roots of spinal nerves, spinal membranes with enclosed cord or cerebrospinal fluid, vessels, fat and areolar tissue. The narrowest part is between T_4 to T_9.

The ligaments are – Supraspinous ligament, interspinous ligament, ligamentum flavum, posterior longitudinal ligament and anterior longitudinal ligament.

Spinal Cord

It is the elongated part of the central nervous system which occupies upper 2/3 of vertebral canal and is 45 cm long. Extent is from upper border of atlas to the upper border of 2nd lumbar vertebra. Superiorly it is continuation of medulla oblongata and below ends in conus medullaris from apex of which filum terminalae descends up to coccyx. The nerve roots passes transversely in early foetal life, then oblique direction so that in adults lumbar and sacral nerves descend vertically up to foramina and this is called as cauda equina. These are bathed in CSF and affected by local anaesthetic agent injected in lumbar area.

Spinal cord is covered by dura mater, arachnoid and pia mater.

The spinal dura mater represents the inner or meningeal layer of cerebral dura mater, the outer endosteal layer covering periosteum lining of vertebral canal which is separated from spinal dura by extradural space. The dural sheath of spinal nerves fuse with the connective tissue lateral to inter-vertebral foramina. A strong fibrous layer forms a tubular sheath attached above to margins of foramina magnum and ending below at lower border of second sacral vertebra. The main fibers are longitudinal so the lumbar puncture needle should be introduced with its bevel facing caudal or cephalic rather than upwards or downwards.

Arachnoid mater is thin sheath closely attached to the dura mater. It surrounds cranial and spinal nerves at their points of exit from skull and vertebral canal.

Pia mater is separated from arachnoid by subarachnoid space containing cerebrospinal fluid and here local anaesthetic solutions are injected. It ends as a prolongation, filum terminalae attached to tip of coccyx.

Spinal segments

Spinal cord is divided into segments by the pairs of spinal nerves arising from it. There are 31 pairs as 8 cervical, 12 thoracic, 5 lumbar, 5 sacral and 1 coccygeal. The nerve roots within dura have no epidural sheath and are easily affected by local anaesthetic solutions.

Spinal nerves

Anterior root is efferent and motor. Sympathetic pre-ganglionic axons arise from cells in inter-medio-lateral horn of spinal cord from $T_1 - L_2$. The blockade of these fibers influences supply to endocrinal glands and to surgical stress.

Posterior root is larger than anterior root. All the afferent impulse from the whole body including viscera pass to posterior roots. These convey the sensation of pain, touch, thermal, deep tendon, joints, bone, afferent from viscera and vasodilator fibers.

The anterior and posterior roots with its covering of pia, arachnoid an dura mater, cross the extradural space and unite in inter-vertebral foramina to form main spinal trunks which soon divides into anterior and posterior primary divisions or mixed nerves. These are blocked secondarily by spinal analgesia.

Analgesic drugs affect autonomic, sensory and motor fibers in that order, fibers which block easily hold the drug for more time, thus sensory block lasts longer than motor and usually ascends two segments higher up in the cord than motor block.

Segmental levels

- Perineum : S_1–S_4
- Inguinal region : L_1
- Umbilicus : T_{10}
- Subcostal arch : T_6–T_8
- Nipple line : T_4–T_5
- 2nd Intercostal space – T_2
- Clavicle : C_3–C_4
- The skin above the nipple line has double innervations from C_3–C_4 and from T_2, T_3 and T_4.

Segmental level of spinal reflexes

- Epigastric : T_7 – T_8
- Abdominal : T_9 – T_{12}
- Cremastric : L_1 – L_2
- Planter : S_1 – S_2
- Knee jerk : L_2 – L_4
- Ankle jerk : S_1 – S_2
- Anal sphincter : S_4 – S_5

8

Regional Anaesthesia

Regional anaesthesia term was first time used by Harvey Cushing in 1901, to describe pain relief by nerve block. E. A. Rovenstine applied technique and advanced the science of therapeutic and diagnostic nerve blocks.

Regional anaesthesia is the anaesthesia of an anatomical part produced by the application of a chemical, capable of blocking conduction in the nerve tissue associated with that part. The functional derangements are reversible.

Theories of Impulse conduction

The nerve membrane consists of bimolecular frame work of phospholipid molecules associated with a globular protein mosaic. A specific gate controls non-specific channels, sodium and potassium, which is voltage dependent. Myelinated nerves are protected by the myelin sheath, which act as an insulation. The local anaesthetic solution prevents depolarization of nerve membrane. As the concentration increases, the height of the action potential is reduced, firing threshold is elevated, the spread of impulse conduction is slowed and refractory period is prolonged. Thus nerve conduction is completely blocked.

The local anaesthetic exert their effect by binding to internal mouth of the sodium channel.

The site of action of local anaesthetic drugs is at the surface membrane of cells of excitable tissues. In Myelinated nerve the site of action is the node of Ranvier. Local anaesthetic drugs are lipoid soluble bases penetrating lipo-protein cell membranes in the non-ionized state.

The blocking quality of local anaesthetic depends on its potency, latecy, nerve diameter, local pH, diffusion rate and concentration of drug, duration of action and regression time.

Methods of Regional anaesthesia

1. Simple topical application at the operative site

- Infiltration analgesia
- Field block.
- Nerve block or conduction anaesthesia
- Refrigeration anaesthesia
- Intravenous Regional anaesthesia
- Surface anaesthesia
- Central Neural blockade

All regional blocks should be preferentially preceded with premedication on humanitarian grounds. The objectives are -

- Sedation with Barbiturates
- Narcotic analgesics to minimize technical discomfort
- Anti-histaminic to protects against allergic response
- Anti-cholinergic for protection against reflex responses
- Some features of Regional anaesthesia are –
- Minimal instrumentation
- One can explain the patient about procedure
- Proper preparation
- Minimum mental trauma
- Minimum physical injury
- After effects are less than general anaesthesia
- Pulmonary complications are less.

Usual indications of Regional anaesthesia :

- Avoidance of dangers and complications related to general anaesthesia as difficult intubation. Postoperative respiratory complications and problems of muscle relaxants.
- It has high quality of postoperative pain relief.
- The facilities of general anaesthesia are not there.

Relative contraindications of Regional anaesthesia when used alone

- In paediatric patients under age of 10 years.
- In noncooperative and psychologically disturbed patients.
- In patients with neurological disorders.
- Prolonged operative procedures
- When means of resuscitation and general anaesthesia supplementation facilities are not available.
- When transport facilities for patient are not there.

General reasons for failure of block

- Anomalies of nerves – anatomical landmarks are not identifiable.
- Errors in diagnosis
- Knowledge of pain
- Lack of knowledge by operator
- Lack of practice
- Inadequate knowledge of anatomy and application of the block. Wrong block at wrong site.

TECHNIQUES OF REGIONAL ANAESTHESIA

Before any large volume of local anaesthetic is injected the following things should be confirmed :

- An open vein
- Tilting table or trolley
- Means of ventilation, Ambu bag or Boyles' machine

- Oxygen supplementation
- Suction apparatus
- Means of endotracheal intubation
- All emergency drugs
- Intravenous fluid in adequate quantity
- Transport facilities : One should identify the nerves to be blocked ideally with nerve locator or anatomical landmarks or with peripheral nerve stimulator.

A) Topical anaesthesia

Topical anaesthesia is administered by painting gauze swabs as liquid in a spray, as a paste, cream or ointment, as an aerosol, by direct instillation (conjunctiva, nose or trachea)

Usual sites of applications are :
- Upper air passage : 4% Lignocaine
- Nasal cavities : 4% Lignocaine
- External ear : 10% aerosol for paracentasis
- Conjunctiva : 4% Lignocaine
- Perineum and vagina : 10% aerosol Lignocaine
- Urethra : 1–2% Lignocaine jelly
- Open wound : 2–4% instillation

B) Infiltration anaesthesia

It is technique of injecting the anaesthetic agent into the tissues to be cut.

C) Field block

It is injecting of local anaesthetic into the tissues about the periphery of area in which surgeon is going to operate.

D) Conduction anaesthesia

- It is accomplished by depositing a local anaesthetic solution along the course of nerve supplying a region of the body, where

elimination of sensation or motor intervention is required.
- Nerve blocks of trunk
- Epidural block : blocking of nerves in epidural space
- Spinal or subarachnoid block : blocking of nerves is subarachnoid space
- Onset and establishment of block is by diffusion, penetration, distribution and fixation of local anaesthetic solution. Reversal and recovery from block is by absorption, reversal, redistribution, destruction and elimination of drug.

IMPORTANT REGIONAL BLOCKS

I) Brachial Plexus Block

Halsted in 1884, Matas & Crile in 1897 injected the plexus under direct vision. KulenKampff used supra-clavicular technique in 1912 and Petrick modified KulenKampff technique in 1940.

Anatomy

The brachial plexus is formed from the anterior primary divisions of C_5, C_6, C_7, C_8 and T_1. It forms the entire motor and almost entire sensory nerve supply to upper extremity or arm. It receives communicating branches from C_4 and T_2 also.

These nerves unite to form three trunks which lie in neck above the clavicle. The roots pass through the fascia enclosed space between the scalenus anterior and scalenus medius accompanied by subclavian artery, invaginate the scalene fascia to form a neuromuscular space, this fascia the becomes axillary sheath which surrounds the plexus. Thus space can be entered at supraclavicular, inter-scalene, axillary or infra-clavicular level.

Each trunk divides behind the clavicle into anterior and posterior divisions which unite in the axilla to forms the cords. The plexus is broad above and converge to first rib. Anteriorly, there is a skin, superficial fascia, platisma and supraclavicular branch of cervical plexus, deep fascia and external jugular vein. The clavicle is in front of its lower part and scalenus anterior muscle is in front of lower part.

The posterior relations are scalenus medius and long thoracic nerve. Inferiorly first rib where plexus lies between subclavian artery and scalenus medius.

The plexus emerges from the intervertebral foramina and passes between scalenus anterior and scalenus medius. At this point, it receives a gray ramus from middle cervical ganglion. 7th and 8th nerves each receives gray ramus from the inferior cervical ganglion.

As the plexus converges on the first rib, it is enclosed in a fibrous sheath with scalenus anterior and scalenus medius :

- The upper trunk is formed by anterior rami of C_5 and C_6
- The middle trunk is formed by anterior rami of C_7
- The lower trunk is formed by anterior rami of $C_5 - T_1$

Behind the clavicle, the trunks divide into anterior and posterior divisions.

- The posterior cord is formed by the posterior divisions : C_5-T_1
- The medial cord is formed by lowest anterior divisions : C_8-T_1
- The lateral cord is formed by upper two divisions : C_5-C_7

The branches arise from roots, trunks and cords.

A) Branches from Roots are
  - Nerve to seratus anterior (Bell) -: $C_5, C_6, C_7.$
  - Dorsalis scapulae : C_5
  - Longus cervices : C_5-C_8
  - Three scalene : C_5-C_8
  - Nerve to Rhomboidus : C_5
  - Twig to phrenic nerve : C_5

B) Branches from Trunk
  - Suprascapular nerve : $C_5 - C_6$
  - Nerve to Subclavian : $C_5 - C_6$

C) Branches from Cords –
  i) Lateral cord -
  - Nerve to lateral pectoral : $C_5 - \dot{C}_7$

- Lateral head of median nerve : $C_5 - C_7$
- Musculocutaneous : $C_{5, 6, 7}$

ii) Posterior cord :
  - Radial nerve : $C_5 - T_1$
  - Axillary nerve : $C_5 - C_6$
  - Thoraco dorsal or nerve to Latismus dorsi : $C_{6, 7, 8}$
  - Upper & lower subscapular nerves : $C_5 - C_6$

iii) Medial cord :
  - Medial head of median nerve : $C_8 - T_1$
  - Medial cutaneous nerve of arm : T_1
  - It is related to Scalenus anterior, scalenus medius, first rib, subclavia artery and subclavian vein.

TECHNIQUES OF BLOCKS OR APPROACHES

a) Supraclavicular
b) Inter-scalene or cervical
c) Subclavian (supraclavicular) perivascular technique
d) Axillary approach

1) Supraclavicular approach

In this technique, the patient is either in sitting or lying supine position. The head is rotated to the other side and arm & shoulder depressed. A wheel is raised 1 cm above the mid point of clavicle lateral to pulsation of subclavian artery.

Needle is inserted inwards and downwards so that it is pointing to spine of 2nd to 4th thoracic vertebrae, when paraesthesia is felt, the solution is injected. It can be blocked after hitting the first rib with slight withdrawal after that. The depth is about 1.2–2.5 cm. Analgesia is rapid in onset and the block settles within 20 minutes. A feeling of warmth and pin & needles precedes analgesia, motor paralysis follows analgesia. 1.5%–2% Lignocaine hydrochloride with adrenaline or 0.25% Bupivacaine hydrochloride or mixture of two can be used. Horner's syndrome may some times noted and it is also guide for successful block.

Complications

- Paralysis of phrenic nerve
- Injury to subclavian artery
- Pneumothorax
- Drug toxicity
- Postoperative permanent neurological complications, are very rare.

2) Interscalene approach – Cervical

This technique was described by Labat in 1927 and modified by Alon Winnie.

The sheath of brachial plexus can be entered via Interscalene space between anterior and middle scalene muscles at the level of C_6 vertebral spine. The patient lies supine, arms by the sides and head turned to opposite side. C_6 spine level can be identified by palpation of the cricoid cartilage or 6th transverse process (Chassaignac's tubercle). At the edge of the sternomastoid muscle the palpating finger lies on the scalenus anterior muscle and more laterally the groove between the anterior and middle scalene muscles. The needle is inserted perpendicular to skin and passing the external jugular vein advanced until the point is felt to enter the perivascular space by a click. After careful aspiration test, the volume of analgesic solution is injected.

It is indicated in operations on shoulder joint, reduction of Colle's fracture.

3) Subclavian (Supraclavicular) perivascular technique

Here the recumbent patient is asked to turn his head to opposite side and to touch his knees. The tip of administrator's index finger is placed posterior to the lateral border of relaxed sternomastoid at the level of C_6 or cricoid cartilage. The tip of finger moves medially behind the belly of sternomastoid and edged inferiorly. The Interscalene groove is palpated and followed down until the subclavian artery is felt. At this point, a short beveled needle is inserted through the clavicular head of sternomastoid and pushed downwards until it enters perivascular space or by a click as the needle pierces fascia. After aspiration, 20–40 ml of local anaesthetic solution is injected slowly. It spares intercosto-bronchial and medial brachial cutaneous nerves and so needs to be blocked separately.

4) Axillary approach

Hirscheld in 1911 first time used this technique of brachial plexus block. In the axilla, the nerves are enclosed in a fibrous neuromuscular fascial sheath. The median and musculo-cutaneous nerves together with their sensory branches are anterior or anterior-lateral i.e. above and behind the artery, ulnar nerve is inferior, radial nerve is posterio-lateral or below and behind the vessel.

Here the patient lies supine with the arm abducted at a right angle, humerus externally rotated and elbow flexed. A wheel is raised at the highest part of the axilla at which arterial palpation is felt, proximal to the lower border of pectoralis major. The pulsatile vessel is identified and through the wheel 2.5 – 5 cm short beveled needle is inserted until and click identifies insertion into neuromuscular sheath. It is very easy to push the needle too deeply. Local anaesthetic solution, 20 ml of 1 – 2% Lignocaine hydrochloride with adrenaline is injected in each quadrant of the vessel. Here the onset of action is delayed up to 30 minutes. It produces complete analgesia below the elbow joint. It is more advantageous than other approaches, as there are less chances of Pneumothorax, Stellate ganglion block, injury to recurrent laryngeal nerve and phrenic nerve. It is some what difficult to adopt in obese patients. With this approach, continuous brachial plexus block by putting catheter can be possible.

Thus brachial plexus block is most satisfactory method of analgesia for operations as dislocation of shoulder and elbow joint, tendon suture, for manipulations, for suturing lacerations on upper extremity.

Direct injury to brachial plexus is very rare and may be due to lack of support to the blocked limb or stretching of nerves.

II) CERVICAL PLEXUS BLOCK

It is paravertebral cervical analgesia. It is not commonly practiced but can be used for removal of superficial tumors and cysts from the neck.

Cervical plexus is formed by anterior primary divisions of the upper 4 cervical nerves, each one after leaving the intervertebral foramina, passes behind the vertebral artery and lie in the sulcus between the anterior and posterior tubercles of the transverse process of the appropriate cervical vertebra. Each of these four nerves except first, divides into upper and lower branches which forms three loops lateral to transverse processes. The loops are between C_1 & C_2, C_2 & C_3, and C_3 & C_4. The upper loop is directed forwards, the lower 2 backwards. The lower branch of C_4 joins C_5 to form brachial plexus.

The branches are superficial (cutaneous), deep (muscular) and communicating. Superficial branches emerge posterior to the lateral border of the sternomastoid, at its midpoint and these are –

Ascending branches : Lesser occiputal and great auricular and supply skin of occiputo – mastoid region, auricle and parotid.

Transverse branch : Anterior cutaneous nerve supply skin of anterior part of neck between lower jaw and sternum.

Descending branches : lateral, intermediate and medial supraclavicular nerves supply skin of shoulder and upper pectoral region.

The Deep branches are – Phrenic nerve, inferior muscular branches and posterior muscular branches to sternomastoid, levator scapulae, trapezius and scalenus medius.

Communicating branches are – Sympathetic gray rami communications from cervical sympathetic chain, the upper four nerves form superior cervical ganglion, branches to vagus nerve, branch to hypoglossal nerve and descending hypoglossal nerve.

The posterior primary divisions of the cervical nerves supply skin and muscles of the back of neck. The nerve supply of thyroid is from middle and inferior cervical sympathetic ganglion and also supplies the oesophagus, vagus, trachea, recurrent laryngeal nerve and sternomastoid muscle.

Technique of the block

Here, the patient lies supine with shoulder slightly elevated, neck and head extended as for thyroidectomy and head turned away from the side to be blocked. O.5%-1% Lignocaine hydrochloride with adrenaline is injected.

Superficial cervical block is carried out by injecting 20 ml of analgesic solution between skin and muscle along the posterior border of sternomastoid muscle near its mid point (just below the point where it crosses external jugular vein) to block ascending, transverse and descending superficial branches of plexus.

Deep cervical block is achieved by the deposition of analgesic solution just lateral to transverse process of 2nd, 3rd and 4th cervical vertebrae. Here the needle is inserted to a depth of 1.5–2 cm perpendicular to all places of the skin, so that the transverse processes are contacted.

It provides analgesia of the front and back of neck, occipital region, cape-like area over the shoulder up to clavicle, 3rd rib and upper border of scapula posteriorly. Mainly it is indicated for Thyroidectomy, superficial tumors in front of neck.

Complications include – phrenic nerve block, intra-thecal or intra-vascular injection of drug, vagus nerve palsy, recurrent laryngeal nerve palsy (aphonia) and cervical sympathetic block causing Horner's syndrome.

III) WRIST BLOCK

Circumferential infiltration just above palm is carried out during wrist block technique. Here median nerve, ulnar nerve and radial nerve are blocked.

- Median nerve (C_5–T_1) at the wrist joint lies deeply between flexor carpi radialis laterally and palmaris longus and flexor digitorium sublimis medially. Injecting 5 ml of 1% Lignocaine hydrochloride lateral to the tendon of palmaris longus, when hand is dorsi-flexed blocks it. The median nerve supplies the skin of thenar eminence and anterior aspect of lateral three and half fingers together with skin over dorsal aspects of their terminal phalanges.

• Ulnar nerve usually divides above the wrist joint into superficial terminal or palmar mixed and dorsal sensory branches. Superficial branch lies between the flexor carpi ulnaris an ulnar artery. It supplies medial part of palm and palmer aspect of 5th and medial side of ring finger. The sensory branch is blocked by injection lateral to flexor carpi ulnaris. The dorsal branch is blocked by intra-dermal and subcutaneous injection at the level of ulnar styloid process or medial side of flexor carpi ulnaris. It supplies ulnar border of dorsum of hand.

• Radial nerve is sensory nerve of back of lateral part of hand. It accompanies radial artery along the medial border of brachio-radialis, it passes 6–7 cm above the wrist joint beneath the tendon and comes to lie beneath the skin on extensor aspect of lower forearm and wrist. It is blocked by injecting the anaesthetic solution on bone at posterio-lateral aspect and the wrist joint near the base of thumb, lateral to radial artery.

This block is used for operations of hand and minor procedures on palm.

IV) DIGITAL BLOCK OR RING BLOCK

Two palmer or two dorsal nerves supply each digit. With a fine needle, an intra dermal wheal is raised on the dorsum of finger near its base. 2 ml of 1% Lignocaine hydrochloride is injected into the substance of finger between the bone and skin and this is repeated to opposite side. The onset of block is some what delayed. Here adrenaline should not added to local anaesthetic solution. It can be blocked by injecting 5 – 7 ml of solution in the intraosseous space of metacarpal bones, entering from dorsal aspect to palmer skin.

It is used for minor operations on fingers or toes.

V) INTERCOSTAL NERVE BLOCK

Each thoracic nerve after emerging from the inter vertebral foramina lie midway between the transverse processes of two adjacent vertebrae,. The nerve then extends obliquely across the intercostal space to the angle of rib above and is further located in the subcostal groove accompanied by a thoracic vein and artery. It is in order of Vein, Artery and Nerve (VAN). Posteriorly, thoracic nerve lie between the external intercostal muscle and then internal intercostal fascia which separates it from pleura and lungs. Anteriorly, the thoracic nerve lie between the internal intercostal muscle and external intercostal fascia. The lateral cutaneous branches of the intercostal nerves arise in the anterior axillary line. The blocking of nerves beyond the angle of rib is called as Intercostal Nerve Block.

Technique

- **At the angle of ribs :** The nerve becomes relatively superficial, lateral to the erector spinal muscle. The patient lies in the lateral position with his back well arched over the edge of table. At a point where the lower border of 11th rib on the patient's upper side crosses the line, a needle is introduced until it makes the contact with the rib. It is then partially withdrawn and advanced until it slips first the lower border of the rib for 3 mm and 2–3 ml of local anaesthetic solution with adrenaline is injected, then the needle point is slightly advanced and withdrawn so as to surround the nerve with analgesic solution. The intercostal nerve is thus surrounded by a zone of solution as it lies in intercostal groove. Thus 10th to 6th nerves on both sides are injected. It produces complete abdominal field block. It may produce complication as Pneumothorax or some times intra dural injection.

- **At the site of Posterior axillary line :** The block can be given when patient lies in supine position with his arms abducted to right angle. In this position, intercostal nerves are not so deep. The block in mid-axillary line spares the lateral cutaneous nerve. There are chances of haematoma formation.

- **At the mid-axillary line :** Intercostal nerves can be blocked at the level of mid-axillary line in the supine position very effectively

Indications

- Blocking of lower 7 intercostal nerves on each side results in analgesia of anterior abdominal wall from nipple line to pubic bone. It produces analgesia of parietal peritoneum and muscle relaxation of anterior abdominal wall.
- It is used to enable the patient to perform deep breathing postoperatively without any pain.
- To reduce post thoracotomy pain.
- As pain relief in multiple fractures of ribs
- For rib resection in Empyema thoracis.

Complications

Pneumothorax, damage to intercostal vessels, haematoma formation.

VI) INGUINAL BLOCK OR HERNIA BLOCK

Anatomy

- Inguinal canal is 4 cm long and extends from the internal inguinal ring laterally to the external inguinal ring medially. It lies above the inner left of inguinal ligament.
- Internal or abdominal ring is just above the midpoint of the inguinal ligament, which is an opening in the transversalis fascia and just medial to inferior epigastric artery.
- Subcutaneous or external ring lies above and lateral to the pubic crest. It is an opening in the external oblique and through it passes the spermatic cord in male and round ligament in female. These all structures lie lateral to the pubic spine.
- Anterior wall : External oblique, internal oblique in its lateral third part.
- Posterior wall : Fascia transversalis, conjoint tendon in inner

two third and reflected part of inguinal ligament in inner one third and femoral vessels.

- Floor : It is formed by the inguinal ligament
- Roof : It has arching fibers of the conjoint tendon of transverse abdominis and internal oblique muscles.
- The content of inguinal canal are – ilio-inguinal nerve, spermatic cord or round ligament.
- All inguinal hernias are protrusions through the fascia transversalis. An indirect hernia protrudes through the deep inguinal ring, descends into the cord and receives covering from the external spermatic fascia, cremestic muscle and internal spermatic fascia.
- Direct hernia protrudes through the fascia transversalis through triangle of Hesselback, bounded by inferiorly epigastric artery, outer border of rectus and inguinal ligament.
- The nerve supply is from last two thoracic nerves via ilio-hypogastric, ilio-inguinal and genito-femoral nerves.

Technique

Three wheals are made as :
- A finger breadth internal to the anterior superior iliac spine
- Over pubic spine
- 1.5 cm above mid-point of inguinal ligament

At first point, the needle is introduced vertically backwards until, pierce sensation is felt of the aponeurosis of external oblique as click. After aspiration, 20-30 ml local anaesthetic solution is injected, so that ilio-inguinal and ilio-hypogastric nerves are blocked. The solution is injected in three directions and in all layers.

At second point, the local anaesthetic solution is injected intra dermal and subcutaneous layers in the direction of umbilicus. It blocks over lapping branches.

At third point, the needle is inserted perpendicular to skin until it pierces the aponeurosis of external oblique. 20 ml of solution is injected to block the genito-femoral nerve.

Intra dermal and subcutaneous infiltration along the line of incision. In addition, infiltration of peritoneum near the pubic tubercle and Astley Cooper's ligament, co-joint tendon, lateral border of rectus abdominis muscle.

It is indicated in slim, poor risk patients posted for laprotomy, to avoid risk of general anaesthesia and subarachnoid block.

To reduce the risk of aspiration in strangulated hernia.

For postoperative pain relief.

It is contraindicated in obesity and un-cooperative patients.

VII) CIRCUMCISION – FIELD BLOCK

The sensory supply of penis is derived from the terminal branches of the internal pudendal nerves. The dorsal nerve of penis travel beneath the pubic bone, one on each side of mid line, lying just above dorsal surface of corpus cavernosum. The skin at the base is supplied by ilio-inguinal and genito-femoral nerves. The posterior scrotal branches of perineal nerves run to ventral surface and fraenum, so here four nerves have to be blocked.

An intra dermal and subcutaneous ring wheal is raised around the base of penis. The dorsal nerve is blocked on each side by injecting 5 ml local anaesthetic solution into dorsum just below but not so deep to the symphysis, so that needle is against corpus cavernosum. For ventral injection, penis is pulled upwards and 2 ml of solution is injected near the base into groove formed by corpus cavernosum and corpus spongiosum. Infiltration of 5 ml solution into each dorsal nerve provides good postoperative analgesia. Adrenaline addition to local anaesthetic is contraindicated in this block. Lignocaine hydrochloride spray or jelly is applied topically for postoperative pain relief.

VIII) ANKLE BLOCK

Subcutaneous and intra dermal weal is raised circumferentially around ankle joint above medial malleolus.

Deep peroneal (Anterior tibial) is blocked by inserting a needle midway between the most prominent points of the medial and lateral malleolus, on the circular line of infiltration in front of ankle joint. It is directed medially towards the anterior border of medial malleolus and local anaesthetic solution is injected between bone and skin. Common peroneal nerve can be blocked ate the neck of fibula where it can be rolled over, 10–15 ml of solution is injected.

Superficial peroneal (musculo-cutaneous nerve) is a branch from the common peroneal nerve, can be blocked above the ankle joint by subcutaneous weal extending from the front of tibia to the lateral malleolus. It supplies dorsum of foot.

Sural nerve : It is the terminal branch of the femoral nerve and accompanies the long subcutaneous vein below and posterior to the lateral malleolus to supply the outer part of the foot and heal. It is blocked by subcutaneous infiltration between the tendoachalis and the prominence of the lateral malleolus using 5–10 ml local anaesthetic solution.

Saphenous nerve : It is the terminal branch of femoral nerve and accompanies the long Saphenous vein, anterior to the medial malleolus where it can be blocked by injection of 10 ml of solution. It supplies an area of skin just below and above medial malleolus.

Tibial Nerve : It passes behind medial malleolus to divide into medial and lateral planter nerves after giving off the medial calcaneal branch. With the patient in prone position, it is blocked by 10 ml of solution injected through point on the circular weal just internal to the tendo-achilles, deep to the flexor reticulum near palpable posterior tibial artery. The needle is inserted forwards and slightly outwards toward the posterior aspect of the tibia. It gets at least 10 minutes for setting of block.

IX) STELLATE GANGLION BLOCK
(CERVICO-THORACIC SYMPATHETIC BLOCK)

Sympathetic block is most commonly carried out in the neck called a Stellate Ganglion block. Stellate ganglion is formed by the fusion of lower three cervical ganglia with first thoracic ganglion. It is irregular is size and position, 1–3 cm long and may differ on either side. With proper injection at perfect site, middle cervical, Stellate and 2nd, 3rd and 4th thoracic ganglia and rami are blocked.

The cervical sympathetic chain and its three ganglia lie in front of the head of first rib and 7th cervical and 1st thoracic transverse process just below the subclavian artery and origin of vertebral artery. It lies posterior to carotid sheath on longus colli and longus cervicis muscles. It is anterior to 8th cervical and 1st thoracic nerves, paraesthesia involving these nerves can be obtained. On th right side, apex of lung and dome of pleura are in anterior relations and on the left side these structures are some what lower. Vaso-constrictor fibers pass from the Stellate and other cervical sympathetic ganglia to a plexus around internal carotid artery. It gives gray rami to the 7th and 8th cervical nerves, gives origin to inferior cervical cardiac nerve and supplies vessels in the vicinity. It may have communication to vagus nerve. Post-ganglionic sympathetic fibers are distributed to the arm with somatic nerves of the brachial plexus and are distributed from them to vessels supplying vaso-constrictor impulses.

Technique

Stellate ganglion block is performed on a patient with an increased bleeding time or decreased time may result is large haematoma in the deep planes of neck.

Para-tracheal approach

Here the patient lies supine, chin forward and neck extended with a pillow to opposite side. A weal is raised 2 finger breadth lateral to the supra sternal notch and similar distance above clavicle which is on the medial border of sternomastoid over lying transverse process of 7th cervical vertebra. The position can be checked by palpating the tubercle of Chassaignac and cricoid cartilage, both are at 6th cervical transverse process. A fine 5–8 cm needle is inserted directly backwards through a weal, while downward and backward pressure is exerted on the sternomastoid to draw the muscle and carotid sheath laterally. When the contact is made with C_7 bone the needle is withdrawn 0.5–1 cm so that its point lies in front of the longus colli muscle and after careful aspiration for blood and CSF, 15 – 20 ml of local anaesthetic solution is injected. When deposited correctly, it will diffuse up and down in the fascial plane and will block the ganglia and rami from $C_2 - T_4$. The block settles within 30 minutes when Horner's syndrome and vasodilatation of arm results.

The other approaches are – anterior approach, lateral approach, and posterior approach or tissue displacement method.

Signs of successful block

- Horner's syndrome : miosis, enophthalmos and ptosis
- Flushing of cheek, face, neck and arm : increase in temperature
- Flushing of conjunctiva and sclera
- Anhydrosis of the face and neck
- Increase in lacrimation
- Stiffness of nostrils (Guttmann's sign)
- Muller's syndrome : injection of tympanic membrane and feeling of warmth in face
- It can be assessed by Cobalt blue and sweat loss, which are more informative than the sympathetic – galvanic response.

Indications

It is indicated to control the tone of intra-cranial vessels.
- To treat Quinine blindness, acute deafness
- To treat acute pain due to Herpes zoster ophthamicus
- Trigeminal neuralgia
- Accidental intra-arterial injection of Thiopentone
- Raynouds' disease : thromboangitis obliterans
- Electrical burns

Complications

- Pleural shock
- Perforation of oesophagus due injury of needle
- Intrathecal injection causing total spinal block
- Intra-vascular injection after accidental injury to vertebral artery
- Pneumothorax

- Rarely cardiac arrest
- Injury to recurrent laryngeal nerve and hoarseness of voice
- Phrenic nerve palsy
- Brachial plexus block
- Extradural or epidural block
- Mediastinitis
- Intercostal neuralgia
- Spilling over of the local anaesthetic solution during brachial plexus block via supra-clavicular route can accidentally block it.
- Bilateral block in one sitting is contraindicated.

IX) INTRAVENOUS REGIONAL ANAESTHESIA (BIER'S BLOCK)

August Bier in 1908 established the effectiveness of local anaesthetic solutions introduced intravenously and localized by tourniquets to produce extensive block.

Mechanism

Local anaesthetics administered intravascularly have a direct action on blood vessel walls and produce vasodilatation. The agent diffuses into tissue and produces anaesthetic block of small nerve fibers and nerve endings. There is a greater localization of the anaesthetic agents in traumatized tissues which is 6 – 8 times greater than in normal tissues. It is due to ease of diffusion from broken capillaries.

Technique

Preliminary measurement of blood pressure establishes the systolic blood pressure and enables the patient to feel the pain of inflated cuff. Localization of an anaesthetic agent to an extremity region is achieved in four steps :

- An intravenous canula or catheter is inserted into a vein distal to the operative site, usually at the back of hand.
- Production of ischemic limb : by elevation of extremity for 2–

3 minutes or by milking blood by means of an Esmarch or Martin bandage, wrapped from the distal portion of the limb toward the proximal part.

- Tourniquet application : The tourniquet cuff is placed at the proximal end of the limb well above the surgical site. Then the cuff is inflated to a level above systolic pressure to prevent re-entry of blood into the limb.
- Injection of a dilute solution of a local anaesthetic through the placed needle or catheter. There may appear tourniquet discomfort within 15–20 minutes due to tightness or paraesthesia.
- Modified or two cuff Technique : It was introduced to reduce tourniquet discomfort. Two tourniquet cuffs are applied close together well above the operative site. After producing ischemia of the limb, the upper or proximal cuff is inflated initially and lower cuff remains deflated, when tourniquet discomfort becomes significant, the lower cuff is inflated followed by deflation of upper cuff. As the lower cuff is in an anaesthetized area, little or no discomfort is experienced and produces good analgesia.

Dosages

The volume of local anaesthetic solution must be sufficient to fill the vascular bed and concentration must be sufficient to produce anaesthesia. Here, large volume of low concentration of local anaesthetic agent is used. The anaesthetic solution is used to replace blood in vascular bed to be anaesthetized. It is thus volume technique and depends on the vascular volume of the extremities. Average dose for upper extremity is 170 ml and for lower extremity is 300 ml.

Dose of 0.3 mg/kg of 0.5% Lignocaine hydrochloride is used. 40–50 ml dose is injected at one time.

As the venous system is a one-way flow system due to the valves, an anaesthetic solution injected into a superficial vein travels proximally from the site of injection to the level of inflated tourniquet. Initially, the solution fills large superficial veins. As the full volume of solution is introduced it concentrates in the region particularly anterior part. The small veins in muscles, deep veins and perforating veins are filled later. After filling the various channels, main nerve trunks are near by, smaller vascular channels take the agent to the core of nerve trunks. In the core, anaesthetic solution diffuses toward the periphery of nerve. It provides anaesthesia for 1 – 2 hours. Tourniquet is released slowly and anaesthetic come into general circulation. The toxic effects are usually seen within 5 – 15 minutes.

It is mainly indicated in superficial and deep operative procedures on upper extremity as orthopaedic procedures, lacerations, suturing, tendon repair, finger contracture can be performed.

One should take precautions as low concentration solutions should be carefully used.

It is contraindicated in allergic disorders to local anaesthetic agents, liver dysfunctions, debilitated and malnourished patients, Sickle cell anaemia, deficient peripheral circulation and myasthenia gravis.

Analgesic drug is released into the circulation in biphasic manner. There is an initial fast release of 30% within 30 minutes.

Toxic signs may be drowsiness twitching, convulsions, bradycardia, hypotension and ECG changes.

Lignocaine hydrochloride is preferred over Bupivacaine hydrochloride due to less chances of toxicity for intravenous regional anaesthesia.

9

Neuromuscular Blocking Agents

Physiology of Neuromuscular Junction

Sir Henry Dale in 1934 has shown that, acetylcholine is responsible for neuromuscular transmission and the effect is blocked by Curare. Then it was shown that, motor nerve liberates acetylcholine from the dense projections in the nerve terminals at myoneural junction as arrival of a nerve impulse.

Acetylcholine crosses the junctional cleft and get fixed at lipoprotein receptos on the junctional folds of the end-plate membrane and permits entry of Sodium which causes sudden depolarization with exit of Potassium from the muscle fiber.

Depolarization passes drug along the membrane of muscle fiber and is final stimulus resulting in contraction of muscle. The released acetylcholine is mean while hydrolyzed by acetyl cholinesterase in the region of motor end plate so the excited muscle comes in refractory state and will not be excited on further stimulus.

Characteristics of depolarizing muscles relaxants

- It causes muscle fasciculations
- Depolarized muscle fibers are un-responsive to other stimuli.
- There is no need of reversing the block
- The block is potentiated by volatile anaesthetic agents (Enflurane, Isoflurane), hypothermia and magnesium

- The block is antagonized by ether, halothane and non-depolarizing muscle relaxants.
- There are chances of phase-II block

Characteristics of non-depolarizing muscle relaxants

- There are no muscle fasciculations
- These are mono–bioquaternary compounds with high electrostatic property and these are hydrophilic.
- The onset of action is relatively slow
- These drugs have characteristic as fade, post-tetanic potentiation or facilitation, exhaustion and depression of twitch response
- The action is potentiated by volatile anaesthetic agents and magnesium
- Action is also potentiated by hypothermia and acidosis.
- These require reversal for weaning with anti-cholinesterase

Classification of muscle relaxants

A) Pharmacological

- Curare like or competitive block – Phase II
- Non-competitive or depolarizing type – Phase I

B) Structure related

- Benzyl isoquinoline – Atracuronium, Cistacuronium, d-tubocurarine
- Steroid nucleus – Pancuronium, Vecuronium

C) According to duration of action

- Long acting – Pancuronium
- Intermediate acting – Atracuronium, Vecuronium
- Short acting – Ropacuronium, Mivacuronium.

SUXAMETHONIUM

- It is bischoline ester of Succinic acid and was introduced by Bovet in 1949. It is depolarizing muscle relaxant acting at the myoneural junction, causing persistent depolarization of motor end plate. The action is similar to acetylcholine on skeletal muscles but the duration of action is somewhat longer.
- It has no actions on central nervous system
- It is white odourless solid, soluble is water, pH is 3.2 to 3.5. Aqueous solutions are relatively stable and can withstand autoclaving.
- It acts on myoneural junction by causing persistent depolarization of the end plate.
- It is degraded by enzymatic hydrolysis in two stages.
- Dose is 1.5–2 mg/kg of body weight or 1 mg/kg/hr infusion

Pharmacological actions

- Autonomic nervous system : Ganglion stimulating action is not so potent, it has mild post-ganglionic cholinergic response causing some decrease in blood pressure which is antagonized by atropine.
- There is no other action on central nervous system as it does not cross blood brain barrier. There is marked increase in spinal fluid pressure which increases within 1 minute and remains elevated up to 3 minutes.
- Cardiovascular System : Most commonly bradycardia may occur. It is noted after single large dose or after subsequent doses as nodal rhythm or extra-systoles. The cardiovascular actions are due to stimulation of autonomic sympathetic ganglia.
- Respiratory System : There is decrease in pulmonary compliance due to muscle fasciculations, some times broncho-constriction noted secondary to histamine release.
- Skeletal muscles : There is pre-ganglionic activation may be due to stimulation of motor neuron terminals with release of

acetylcholine or due to stimulation of the end plate in extrafusal muscle system.

- Action on smooth muscles : It causes some relaxation of smooth muscles of blood vessels, eye ball, ureters, etc.
- Gastro-intestinal tract : There is increase in intra-gastric pressure due abdominal wall muscle fasciculations. It has an opening effect on the cardiac sphincter due to pulling of crura, when stomach is distended, so there is possibility of regurgitation. There is no much increase in intra-gastric pressure particularly in paediatric patients.
- There is limited histamine release after Suxamethonium.
- It does not crosses placental barrier, so there is no effect on foetus and new born.
- After intravenous administration, the drug is destroyed by pseudo-cholinesterase. The onset of action in quicker within 1–2 minutes and duration of action is for 3–5 minutes. Some times it may be for 10–12 minutes.
- The neuromuscular block is terminated by its diffusion away from end plate into extra-cellular fluid compartment.
- The duration of action may be prolonged due to low levels of pseudo-cholinesterase as in liver diseases, severe anaemia, hyperpyrexia, cardiac failure, uremia, or cholinesterase inhibitors as Neostigmine, Pyridostigmine, Echothiopate, Cyto-toxic drugs or Organo-phosphorus compounds.
- Normal levels of pseudo-cholinesterase enzyme is 80–120 IU/100 ml. Dibucaine number determines the percentage inhibition of the enzyme.

Clinical uses

- For endotracheal intubation during general anaesthesia.
- As an infusion for muscle relaxation in balanced technique of anaesthesia and dose is 0.1 mg/kg/min.
- For electro-convulsive therapy
- During crash induction of anaesthesia in emergency
- As a muscle relaxant in short surgical procedures without

endotracheal intubation as orthopaedic manipulations, anal dilatation, cervical dilatation, etc.

Contraindications

- Anticipated difficult endotracheal intubation
- Extremes of age
- Known case of low levels of pseudo-cholinesterase enzyme
- Liver disease
- Kidney dysfunction
- Critically ill, malnourished and cachexia patients
- Motor neuron disease
- Hyperkalamia due to any cause
- Raised intra-cranial tension due to any cause
- Malignant hyperthermia
- Known sensitivity to the drug
- Means of endotracheal intubation and resuscitation are not available

Complications

- Prolonged apnoea due to :
    - Atypical pseudo-cholinesterase
    - Dehydration and electrolyte imbalance
    - Low levels of pseudo-cholinesterase
    - Excessive formation of succinyl monocholine
    - Phase II block
- Increase in intra-occular pressure
- Increase in intra-gastric pressure and regurgitation
- Muscle pain
- Histamine release – bradycardia and hypotension
- Increase in salivary and gastric secretions
- Increase in serum potassium level and Hyperkalamia
- Hypothermia increases the intensity of block
- Some times hypertension

Drug interaction

- Potentiation of block and prolongation of action in cases with low levels of pseudo-cholinesterase levels as with Echothiopate drops, Procaine, Cytoxic drugs, Organo-phosphorus compounds, tacrine, etc.
- Pitocin or Oxytocin, it alters the sensitivity of the end plate to depolarization and it prolongs the effect.
- Ganglion blocking drugs compete with acetylcholine at neuromuscular junction and potentiate the action of non-depolarizing muscle relaxants and antagonize the action of depolarizing drugs.
- Quinidine prolongs the effect by decreasing end plate sensitivity to transmitter
- Neostigmine and anti-cholinesterase drugs delay the hydrolysis of drug.
- Lithium increases the duration of action
- Propanidid prolongs the duration of action due to same pathway of hydrolysis.

d-TUBOCURARINE

Curare was firstly used as arrow poison by the tribes residing in South Africa. It was obtained from the bark of various species of Strychinos and from Chondrodendron tomentosum. It was transported in bamboo tubes and so named as tubocurarine. Claude Bernard discovered its action on neuro-muscular junction and was isolated by King in 1935. Griffith and Jhonstone used it for first time in 1940 for clinical anaesthesia.

It produces muscle relaxation by competitive inhibition of the neuromuscular junction. It combines with the end plate receptors and there by prevents release and entry of acetylcholine thus obstructs reaching to receptor substance. Thus it produces non- depolarizing type of block.

Curare is generic form which contains Intocostrin (crystalline tubocurarine), d-tubocurarine chloride, dimethyl tubocurarine.

It blocks the impulses from medulated cholinergic motor fibers to striated muscle cells. It also block the synaptic transmission at autonomic ganglia i.e. between pre-ganglionic cholinergic fibers and post-ganglionic cell body.

Following intravenous administration, there is rapid redistribution of the drug and 30–50% binds with globulin part of plasma proteins. The unbound drug is distributed through out extra-cellular compartment within 20 minutes. It is found in liver up to 6 hours but is has little effect on liver and kidney functions. It is mostly excreted through urine and 10–20% excreted via bile.

Dose : 0.3 mg/kg or 0.5 mg/kg for muscle relaxation during general anaesthesia.

Pharmacological actions

1. **Central Nervous system :** It does not cross blood brain barrier but it has some indirect actions on central nervous system.

2. **Cardiovascular system :** In clinical doses there is no effect on circulation of the patient. Relatively in high doses, there is decrease in blood pressure secondary to ganglion blocking action, smooth muscle relaxation and decrease in venous return. The hypotension may be due to some histamine release attributed to drug. It has positive inotropic action.

3. **Respiratory system :** The actions on respiratory system are related to paralysis of respiratory muscles, there is broncho-constriction due action on smooth muscles and histamine release. There is increase in tone of bronchodilators muscles following histamine release. The increase in bronchiolar tone increases airway resistance to inflation of lungs and decrease in pulmonary compliance. There are chances of increase of thick tenacious secretions due to histamine release and results in blockage of airway passage.

4. **Autonomic nervous system :** It depresses the ganglionic transmission. It does not interfere with acetylcholine formation by pre-ganglionic terminals but prevents acetylcholine from reaching the effectors substance of post-ganglionic cell. This action is antagonized by neostigmine. The ganglionic blocking action on parasympathetic ganglia is more intense than

sympathetic system. Salivary secretions and intestinal movements are more blocked.

5. **Gastro-intestinal tract :** In therapeutic doses, it relaxes smooth muscles of intestinal tract. It decreases the tone and motility of gut.

There are no effects on kidney and liver functions.

It does not crosses placental barrier.

Indications

- Clinically it is used to produce muscle relaxation during balanced technique of anaesthesia. The onset of action is within 2–3 minutes, with peak effect at 4–8 minutes and duration of action up to 20–30 minutes. The action can be easily reversed with neostigmine.
- It is particularly useful in poor risk patients
- The dose requirement is more in patients with liver diseases.
- It is not contraindicated in liver and kidney diseases.
- Now a day it is not available.

GALLAMINE TRIETHIODIDE

- It is synthetic non-depolarizing muscle relaxant introduced by Bovet in 1947. It acts by preventing acetylcholine from reaching the end plate by competing for the receptor substance.
- Dose is 2–2.5 mg/kg, the onset of action starts within 2 minutes and duration is up to 20–25 minutes.
- The action is antagonized by neostigmine effectively.
- It has no direct action on myocardium. There is increase in pulse rate and blood pressure, mediated through vagal blocking action.
- There is very little histamine release.
- It readily crosses placental barrier and so not used during caesarian section.
- It is totally excreted via kidney so contraindicated in severe renal disorders.

- There is no effect on liver functions and can be used in patients with liver diseases without ant side effects.
- Volatile anaesthetic agents like Ether and Halothane potentiate the action.
- Usually it is used as muscle relaxant during balanced technique of anaesthesia.

PANCURONIUM BROMIDE

- It is bis-quaternary amino steroid, which is not having any hormonal activity. Bernard and Reid introduced it in 1967.
- It is non-depolarizing type of muscle relaxant, which is 5 times more potent than d-tubocurarine.
- Dose is 0.1 mg/kg and elimination half-life is 14.5 minutes.
- The onset of action is within 1–3 minutes and duration lasts for 25–40 minutes.
- It does not cross blood brain barrier, so there are no direct actions on central nervous system.
- There is mild vagolytic action on myocardium but there is no ganglion blocking action. It may produce mild tachycardia with some increase in blood pressure. These actions are attributed to its vagolytic and sympathomimetic effect. There is increase in cardiac output due to increase in heart rate.
- There is very little placental transfer of drug into foetal circulation.
- There is no histamine release with this and so hypersensitivity reactions are rare. It is well tolerated by sensitive patients also, like bronchial asthma.
- It has no direct actions on liver and kidney functions.
- After intravenous administration, 87% of drug binds with albumin part of plasma proteins. It has no cumulative effect.
- Most of the drug is metabolized in liver. After intravenous administration, 30% of drug is eliminated in urine within 8 hours and 24% is excreted in bile. It has 3–H–Pancuronium as metabolite which is 50% active as that of parent drug Pancuronium bromide.

- In patients with renal disorders, excretion via bile is increased and vice versa.
- As it has rapid onset of action, it can be used for endotracheal intubation when Suxamethonium is contraindicated or not available.
- Now it is most commonly used non-depolarizing muscle relaxant for balanced technique of anaesthesia, for endotracheal intubation, in patients with cardiovascular disorders, shock states, critically ill patients, extremes of age, liver disorders, liver diseases, electrolyte imbalance, etc.
- As such it has no contraindications and also there are no dreadful side effects or complications with it.

VECURONIUM

- It is an androstanyl derivative of acetylcholine and a potent non-depolarizing neuromuscular blocking agent with medium duration of action.
- It is mono quaternary ammonium compound. It is 4.4 times more potent than Atracuronium and slightly more potent than Pancuronium.
- Dose is 0.1 mg/kg which produces satisfactory endotracheal intubating conditions within 90 seconds. It can be given in 0.15 – 0.2 mg /kg for better muscle relaxation.
- Inhalational anaesthetic agent like Halothane potentiates the duration of action. The duration of action is approximately 15–20 minutes.
- It dissolves in water and stable for 24 hours at room temperature and for days together at 4°C, pH of solution is 4.
- It can be given as infusion in dose of 1¼ gm/kg/min, hepatic degradation is 20–30%, biliary excretion is 40–60% (unchanged) and renal excretion is 15–20%. It is re-distributed and rapidly cleared from plasma.
- There is less cumulative effect on repeated doses.
- Metabolism is affected in severe hepatic disorders.

- There is no histamine release. Some times hypersensitivity reactions are noted with it.
- It has no ganglionic blocking or vagal blocking action and without sympathomimetic effect. There is no change in pulse rate and blood pressure.
- It does not cross placental barrier and so can be used in caesarian section.
- Infants and neonates are resistant to its effect as compared to adults.
- The neuromuscular block is potentiated in presence of metabolic acidosis. Alkaline medium accelerates decomposition of the drug.
- The neuromuscular block may produce spontaneous recovery without specific antidote but usual reversal with Neostigmine is always carried out.

ATRACURONIUM

- It is bisquaternary ammonium compound is highly specific, competitive neuromuscular blocking agent was synthesized by Stenlake in 1983.
- It is stable at pH above 3.5 and stored at 4°C. temperature.
- It is self destroyed by Hoffmann reaction in the body at pH 7.4 and 37°C. It breaks down to laudanosine and other products, which are devoid of significant neuromuscular and cardiovascular effects.
- It is also destroyed by ester hydrolysis, which is major pathway of elimination. This bypass elimination pathway is active when normal metabolism and excretion is affected as in liver or renal disorders.
- It is one-fifth as potent as Vecuronium.
- Dose is 0.2 mg/kg for muscle relaxation and 0.5 mg/kg for endotracheal intubation and 6–8¼ gm/kg/minute as infusion.
- The onset of action is within 3–5 minutes and duration of action or recovery time is 20–35 minutes.

- The action is potentiated by volatile anaesthetic agents, metabolic acidosis and decomposed in alkaline medium.
- There is little histamine release with it.
- It is devoid of any sympathetic stimulation, vagolytic or ganglion blocking action. There is no significant change in pulse rate and blood pressure so it is cardiovascular stable. Bradycardia mat be noted when Atropine is not given as premedication or along with Halothane anaesthesia.
- Other non-depolarizing muscle relaxants recently introduced in anaesthesia practice are :
  - Alcuronium   - Fazadinium
  - Dacuronium   - Cistacuronium
  - Mivacuronium   - Rocuronium
  - Doxacuronium   - Pipecuronium
  - Rapacuronium

These all are under trials, costly and not available easily in India.

NEOSTIGMINE METHYL SULPHATE

Aesctimann of Reinert synthesized neostigmine methyl sulphate in 1931. It is twice as potent as Physiostigmine.

- It prevents normal hydrolysis of acetylcholine, so it allows acetylcholine to accumulate at neuromuscular junction.
- It is partly broken down by serum cholinesterase and partly excreted unchanged by the kidneys. It binds to the esteratic sub site of cholinesterase with its carbonate group.

Pharmacological actions

- It is quaternary ammonium compound so does not cross blood brain barrier.
- It increases both muscarinic and nicotinic effects of acetylcholine. The muscarinic actions are due to stimulation of the effectors organs of post-ganglionic para-sympathetic nerve endings in sweat glands and uterus. The muscarinic

effects include bradycardia, hypotension, profuse salivary and bronchial secretion, bronchospasm, stimulation of smooth muscles of viscera, etc.

- Nicotinic actions of Neostigmine are due to stimulation of pre-ganglionic autonomic fibers, adrenal medulla and motor nerves of skeletal muscles.
- It prolongs and increases local depolarization produced at the end plate by acetylcholine. It may potentiate actions of depolarizing muscle relaxants.
- It may produce fasciculations.
- It itself produces firstly depolarizing type of block and then non-depolarizing type of block when it is not used for reversal.
- Prior administration of Neostigmine prolongs the duration of action of Suxamethonium.
- It does nor cross blood brain barrier as well as placental barrier, so no actions on central nervous system and on foetus.
- Dose is 0.04–0.08 mg/kg diluted given slowly to have maximum beneficial effects for reversal of non-depolarizing type of block. The onset of action is within 3–5 minutes. It is always given along with Atropine 0.02 mg/kg or with Glycopyrolate 0.2 mg. The duration of action may be for 1 hour.

Clinical Uses

- For reversal of non-depolarizing type of neuromuscular block.
- For reversal of Phase II block after Suxamethonium.
- In treatment of myasthenia gravis
- In diagnosis of neuromuscular disorders.
- In treatment of snake bite.
- Untoward effects are – increased salivation, excessive bronchial secretions, increased intestinal motility, bradycardia, shifting of pacemaker, conduction defects. So Atropine should be used along with Neostigmine.
- Respiratory acidosis and metabolic alkalosis may impair the

actions of Neostigmine. Enflurane slows the reversal of neuromuscular block with Neostigmine.

- Over doses may cause restlessness, weakness, muscular twitching, sweating, increased salivation, pin-point pupils, abdominal colic, hypotension and even cardiac arrest.

- Massive over doses of muscle relaxants, electrolyte imbalance, hypokalamia, respiratory acidosis, Quinidine, local anaesthetic agents, antibiotics may interfere with normal reversal of non-depolarizing block with Neostigmine.

GALLANTHAMINE HYDROBROMIDE

- This alkaloid is extracted from snow drop bulb and has been used in the Eastern Europe in the treatment of reversal of the neuromuscular block, or disorders. It was reported to be an antagonist to non-depolarizing muscle relaxants in 1962.

- Chemically, it is a phenantridine derivative and structurally related to morphine. It acts as anti-cholinesterase with about 1/10 potency of Neostigmine.

- Both plasma cholinesterase and pseudo-cholinesterase are inhibited by the action of this drug. There is no depression of neuromuscular transmission like Neostigmine with it

- It has property that non-depolarizing drugs action is antagonized and the action of depolarizing drugs is potentiated. The degree of potentiation of Suxamethonium is less than that of Hydroflauronium.

- After Gallanthimine injection along with Suxamethonium, it is accompanied by more fasciculations and more bradycardia if given alone

- The muscarinic side effects are less than with that of Neostigmine but Atropine should be given along with it

- The dose is 5–10 mg intravenously. Additional doses up to 20–30 mg may be needed to produce complete reversal of the non-depolarizing block. With larger doses, persistent antagonism is achieved with some analeptic and stimulating action

- The duration of action is up to 2 hours and thus it provides the persistent antagonism
- Only mild muscarinic effect is noted. So small doses of Atropine are given to minimize salivation, mild decreases in pulse rate and blood pressure
- It itself can cause respiratory depression of central origin due to Morphine like action. It is mainly due to the structural similarity of Morphine which provides competitive action like morphine at the receptor site.

10

Monitoring During Anaesthesia

Administration and conduction of anaesthesia is not only the duty of anaesthesiologist but it is keeping the safety of the patient through out intraopertaive and early postoperative period, irrespective of the surgical procedure performed on the patient with any technique of anaesthesia. This is called as monitoring in the patient.

There are some guide lines or pre-requisites for monitoring of patient :

- One must monitor only one patient at one time.
- Monitor the patient from starting i.e. preferably from preanaesthesia check up, induction of anaesthesia, through out intraopertaive period till the patient is shifted to recovery room or surgical intensive care unit or in the ward.
- Clinical monitoring is more important than instrument monitoring.
- Monitor all the patient thoroughly in spite of the technique of anaesthesia as only sedation, local anaesthesia, regional blocks or balanced general anaesthesia. No operative procedure would be carried out in absence of expert anaesthesiologist or he may be only asked to stand by.
- Carefully monitor the patients of extremes of age (neonates, infants and geriatric), major operative procedures, emergency

operative procedures and patients with associated mild to severe systemic medical disorders.

- Always there should be one assistant during monitoring particularly in above situations.
- Take help of various monitors as additional helping hand and do not totally depend up on the monitors.

Usually monitoring is performed by two ways –

- Clinical monitoring
- Instrument monitoring

Clinical Monitoring

- Colour of skin and blood for oxygenation
- Pulse for – rate, rhythm, volume for cardiac performance or peripheral circulation
- Blood pressure (systolic and diastolic) for peripheral circulation
- Respiratory movements for adequacy of ventilation
- Movements of reservoir bag for respiratory efforts
- Temperature of skin for body temperature, circulatory status and fluid balance.
- Urine out put for kidney function and control over in put.
- Excessive sweating or perspiration, lacrimation for depth of anaesthesia
- Muscle tone or movements for muscle relaxation or need for supplementary dose of relaxants for inadequacy or regional block.
- Pupils for depth of anaesthesia or stage of surgical anaesthesia with Ether anaesthesia or state of cerebral circulation
- Awareness during anaesthesia
- Blood loss
- Central venous pressure by observing filling of jugular veins
- Surgeon's satisfaction.
- Clinical monitoring is carried out with the help of hands, eyes, ear or nose as sensory monitors of touch, vision, hearing and smell.

- Basic instruments for monitoring a patient
- Circulation–non-invasive B.P. monitor, ECG and Pulsoximeter
- Respiration–IPPV, airway pressure, Ventilatory volume, capnography, Pulsoximeter, disconnection alarms
- Metabolic status–Capnography, blood glucose, acid base balance
- Neuromuscular transmission–nerve stimulator

Basic instrumental monitoring of anaesthesia machine

- Oxygen failure alarms
- Airway pressure monitoring
- Ventilatory failure alarms

Additional instrumental monitoring

- Urine out put measurement
- Body temperature monitoring
- Pulmonary artery catheterization
- Intra-arterial blood pressure monitoring
- Blood gas analysis
- Blood glucose, electrolytes, clotting time
- Non-invasive cardiac out put measurement, ECG, metabolism and oxygenation, awareness, etc.
- Clinical monitoring is more important than any instrumental monitoring. Monitoring of vital parameters as pulse, blood pressure, pain, reflexes, adequacy of level of anaesthesia, temperature, urine out put, pupils, heart sounds, respiration, cyanosis, resistance to ventilation, colour of skin, colour of blood, etc should be carried out irrespective of technique of anaesthesia.

Monitoring during anaesthesia

- One should see that, the level of operating table is whether horizontal or not. It should not have head or foot tilt as it interferes with the circulation in patient. Foot drop decrease the venous return and may result in hypotension. Head down tilt may cause congestion of eyes and head may interfere in brain circulation or chances of hypoxia in severe cases.

- Hand should be at the same level of body or parallel to the operation table and right angle to the extended arms of both sides. The change in position of hands may give traction on nerve plexus or nerves.

- The eyes of the patient should be protected and just closed by cotton pad to avoid drying of conjunctiva. Liquid paraffin should be installed in eyes to avoid this particularly during prolonged operative procedures.

- Monitor intravenous infusion setting for flow as there are chances of obstruction to flow by pressure of body or hands of the surgeon or assistant. It should not go out or extravasations of hypertonic solutions may result in sloughing of skin.

- When the patient is on spontaneous respiration, watch the respiration for adequacy of any obstruction during regional or general anaesthesia, obstruction to ventilation during controlled ventilation due to kinking of the endotracheal tube, corrugated tube, resting on the corrugated tube by surgeon or his assistant, secretions, bronchospasm, etc, There might be resistance to spontaneous due to keeping of instruments on abdomen of the patient or resting of hand on abdomen. If it is noted ask the surgeon to remove the obstructing element.

- Monitor the eye for lacrimation which might be light plane of anaesthesia or further need of analgesic supplement. Monitor for pupillary reaction and size intermittently to note level of anaesthesia particularly during Ether anaesthesia or prolonged operative procedures, blood loss, hypoxia, etc. There might be constricted pupils during light plane of anaesthesia and with high doses of narcotic analgesics. There might be slow dilatation of pupils as effect of hypoxia or very deep planes of Ether anaesthesia or late stages of life. Dryness of conjunctiva is noted due to opening of eyes secondary to muscle relaxants or chemosis may occur due to over transfusion of fluids or raised jugular venous pressure.

- During regional anaesthesia, intermittently awaken the patient to note toxic effects of local anaesthetic agents or drowsiness twitching, convulsions, hypoxia, high level of spinal anaesthesia or total spinal block.

- Monitor the flow of gases Oxygen and Nitrous oxide at flow meter, gauze for exhaustion of cylinders and correct it accordingly by changing the cylinder. Monitor the level of inhalational anaesthetic agents in the bottles for refilling.

- When the patient is on spontaneous respiration, monitor the movements of the reservoir bag which deflates during inspiration and inflates during expiration of the patient by visual impression. During controlled or assisted ventilation observe the feel of reservoir bag and note the resistance which might be due to obstruction secondary to external pressure on the corrugated tube, internally excessive secretions, bronchospasm, pulmonary oedema, etc. and correct these conditions accordingly. The resistance to ventilation due to any cause should be detected early and treated quickly. Note the gurgling sounds in the reservoir bag which the sign of excessive secretions of pulmonary oedema and treat it as medical emergency.

Pulse of the patient

- Always monitor pulse of the patient continuously for presence, rate, rhythm, volume and bilateral equality. Usually the radial pulse at wrist joint is monitored as it is to approach, reliable and easily palpable. When the pulse is not palpable then confirm it on the other hand and then on the major arteries as external carotid or confirm by audibility of heart sound with stethoscope. Absence of pulse on palpation should be considered as medical emergency and treated accordingly and then find out the cause. This may lead to ir-reversible cardiac arrest

- Intraoperatively severe bradycardia or impending arrest may occur –
    - At the induction of anaesthesia, direct myocardial

depression due to intravenous Thiopentone or if Atropine premedication is not given.

- Rarely after bolus dose of Suxamethonium
- At the time laryngoscopy in light plane of anaesthesia or inadequate muscle relaxation.
- During normal endotracheal intubation due to vagal stimulation or forceful laryngoscopy and intubation
- At the time of positioning of patient due to total sympathetic blockade and parasympathetic over activity.
- When tip of endotracheal tube is touching carina
- At the time of incision over body in light plane of anaesthesia
- Orthopaedic manipulations in light plane of anaesthesia
- High level of spinal anaesthesia due blockade of cardiac sympathetics
- As a feature of Bruward Luckhard's reflex during anal dilatation, opening of pleura and peritoneum, mastoid surgery, manipulations at hilum of vital organs due to vaso-vagal stimulation
- Intraopertaive increase in intra-cranial pressure, intra-occular pressure or intra-abdominal pressure and during insufflation of gas in laproscopy
- It may be due to high concentration of Halothane or immediate high concentration of Ethyl chloride spray, when atropine is not mixed with Neostigmine.

• So one must ascertain the bradycardia and treat it immediately either with Atropine 0.01 mg/kg and when there is no response again repeat the same dose. Again if it is not responding then one may try intravenous Isoprenaline 2 mg diluted or lastly temporary or permanent pacemaker. If the bradycardia is not treated in time then it may result in impending cardiac arrest.

• Monitor the pulse for tachycardia in the range of more than 20% - 30% increase from normal basal reading. It may be due to sympathetic stimulation due to any cause as light plane of anaesthesia, systolic hypertension, pre-existing thyrotoxicosis, congestive cardiac failure, left ventricular failure, myocarditis, pulmonary oedema, hypoxia, systemic hypotension due to fluid or blood loss, inadequate carbon dioxide removal, exhausted soda lime, weaning from action of muscle relaxants, etc. Here also one must detect exact cause of tachycardia and mainly correct the causative factor which will automatically treat the tachycardia.

- Bradycardia is more dangerous and need prompt treatment than tachycardia.

- One should see the volume of pulse, whether normal, high volume or low volume. Low volume pulse is the diagnostic feature of hypotension secondary to peripheral circulatory failure or pressure over course of artery.

- High volume pulse may be due to awareness during anaesthesia, inadequate analgesia, hypertension, soda lime exhaustion, increase in intra-occular and intra-cranial pressure, hyperthermia, thyrotoxicosis, etc. The exact cause of high volume of pulse should be noted and treated accordingly.

- See for rhythm of pulse as regular or irregular, if irregular then regularly irregular or irregularly irregular. Irregular pulse or missed beats may be noted due to increase in intra-cranial and intra-occular pressure, soda lime exhaustion, Carbon dioxide retention, ischemic heart disease, various types of heart blocks, sinus arrhythmia, etc. Here one should confirm it and treat it promptly and if needed take opinion of physician.

- All peripheral pulses should be palpated intermittently particularly in patients with ischemic heart disease, patient on anti-coagulant therapy, deep vein thrombosis, varicose veins, vascular surgery, cardio-pulmonary bypass, thrombo-embolic phenomenon, caesarean section, vesicular mole, open heart surgery, valvotomy, patients with liver disease, etc. It should be detected promptly and treated accordingly.

- Blood pressure: (systolic & diastolic) : Monitor systolic blood pressure continuously and systolic with diastolic intermittently at regular intervals. Increase or decrease by 20–30 mm of Hg in systolic blood pressure should be carefully noted and corrected accordingly. There might be severe hypotension at the time of administration of Thiopentone sodium due to direct myocardial depressant action, peripheral vasodilatation, intravenous high dose of Diazepam, during change of position, prone position, lithotomy position, after spinal anaesthesia, some times with epidural block, anaphylactic reactions, vasovagal stimulation in light plane of anaesthesia, neurogenic or haemorhagic shock or iatrogenic cause. Hypotension should be promptly corrected according to the cause.

Intra-operative hypertension may be noted due to light plane of anaesthesia, sympathetic stimulation due to any cause, patient coming out of action of muscle relaxants, raised intra-cranial tension, carbon dioxide retention, soda lime exhaustion, Ketamine anaesthesia, endotracheal tube touching to carina, undiagnosed phaeochromocytoma, need of analgesic supplementation due to prolonged operative procedure, etc. Intra-operative hypertension should be treated immediately to avoid further increase in blood pressure and subsequent complications.

- One should monitor pupillary size and reaction intermittently, particularly when patient is on Ether anaesthesia, very prolonged and major operative procedure, intra-operative severe blood loss, hypotension and then hypoxia or for any untoward effect.

- One should see the body temperature by touch or with temperature monitor which is important in paediatric patients (infants and neonates), emergency operative procedures with infective focus, hyperthermia, thyrotoxicosis. One should note coldness of extremities in severe hypotension due to peripheral circulatory failure, winter season which is also important in neonates and infants. Hypothermia may be noted after rigors, intravenous fluids or cold massive blood transfusion. It can be noted as pilo-errection due to severe shock. The changes in temperature should be treated by counter action as hyperthermia is treated by cold sponging or hypothermia is treated by taking measures of rewarming patients.

- Intermittently one should monitor cyanosis as bluish tinge of nails beds of fingers, lips, colour of blood at the site of operation which might be due to inadequate supply oxygen, Ventilatory inadequacy, bronchospasm, laryngospasm, metabolic acidosis due to any cause, respiratory acidosis, pulmonary oedema due to any cause, exhaustion of soda lime, blood diseases, etc. It should be treated with oxygen supplementation or positive pressure ventilation with 100% oxygen and treat the basic cause.

- Monitor for the movements of extremities as resistance to ventilation indicating wearing of action of muscle relaxants or surgeon may complain of inadequate muscle relaxation

- Monitor the surgeon for what and how operative procedure is being carried out, what assistant is doing, watch for sister's assistance regularly. See the suction apparatus for total amount of suction, whether is it is peritoneal or pleural fluid, whether it is watery, mixed with blood or only blood to note the fluid loss and accordingly correct the fluid loss either with intravenous fluids, crystalloids or colloids and blood whenever necessary.

- Monitor for the colour of the water used by the sister for swabs soaking and how many times it was changed, to note the blood loss in the intraopertaive period.

- Intraoperatively monitor the patient on Pulsoximeter for pulse rate, oxygen saturation, capnography for end tidal CO_2, ECG monitor for changes in pulse rate, rhythm or any other ECG abnormality, invasive blood pressure (systolic and diastolic), central venous pressure and urine output for adequate intravenous fluids and kidney functions.

- All these observations clinical and monitoring devices should be seen intermittently or continuously till the end of operative procedure.

- The course of anaesthesia, changes in vital parameters, intravenous fluids given, urine output, total fluid collection in the suction, all these should be noted either on case paper of the patient or anaesthesia record or Noseworthy cards. This is

. very important for medico-legal view.

- One should monitor for the Surgeon's operative procedure about what he is doing, what is the step of anaesthesia, blood loss, fluid loss, during laprotomy the surgeon is not bothered about for period the coils of intestines are out of the abdomen which will result in fluid loss or dryness of coils. If there is any difficulty, then help the surgeon in completion of the operative procedure.

- One should observe for what step of operative procedure so at the end of operative procedure one has to stop the increments of muscle relaxants so that at proper time one is able to reverse the patient. Again there are some operative procedures where the anaesthesiologist has to be careful about administration of Nitrous oxide (ENT procedures or operations in close cavity) to avoid ill effects of diffusion hypoxia. One has to guide the surgeon in controlling the blood loss, advise about the clamping of big veins to avoid chances of air embolism, pull of mesenteries, prolonged traction or catching in the forceps which may result in necrosis due to obstruction to blood supply.

- One should ask for blood transfusion at proper time and again remind the surgeon about the operative time in very prolonged operative procedures so that un-necessary time lapse will not be there in betterment of patient.

- In patients receiving regional blocks one should also monitor all vital parameters as pulse rate, blood pressure, respiration, adequacy of block, analgesia and muscle relaxation achieved, comfort of the surgeon, complications related to regional block, toxicity of local anaesthetic agent, anaphylactic reactions, requirement of supplementation, etc.

- Under spinal or epidural block, one should monitor for changes in pulse rate as sudden bradycardia, blood pressure as hypotension, level of analgesia, adequacy of sensory block as (good, fair or poor), degree of motor blockade (grade – I,II,III or IV), onset of sensory block, onset of motor block, duration of sensory and motor blockade, duration of operative procedure, incidence of intra-operative and **postoperative** complications as nausea, vomiting, respiratory inadequacy, drowsiness, tremors, involuntary movements, convulsions and unconsciousness, delayed postoperative complications related to technique of anaesthesia as permanent neurological sequalae, etc. All this is monitored intermittently and continuously through out operative procedure and postoperatively in recovery room and wards.

Additional Instrumental Monitoring

- Urine output and temperature monitoring in major surgical procedures
- Pulmonary artery catheterization
- Transthoracic impedence apnoea alarms, intra-arterial blood pressure, intermittent or continuous blood gas analysis, End Tidal CO_2, etc.
- Blood tests – Blood sugar, Electrolytes, Coagulation profile, hormonal assay, Complete blood count, etc.
- Non-invasive monitoring - cardiac output, cerebral electrical activity, Oxygenation, state of awareness.
- The instrumental monitors have their problems of acclimatization, sensing, electrical dis-connection, data interpretation and so clinical monitoring is many times more reliable.

11

Anaesthesia Machine

ANAESTHESIA MACHINE

Boyle's anaesthesia machine is a continuous flow machine used for the administration of inhalational anaesthesia. The machine was introduced by Henry Boyle (Henry Edmond Goskin Boyle) in 1917.

- Originally, Boyle's introduced Nitrous oxide-Oxygen anaesthesia through this machine and it was a two gas system with water tight sight-feed type of flow meter. In 1920, modification was made by incorporating a vaporizing bottle to flow meter. A second vaporizing bottle and bypass controls were added in 1926.
- Plunger device in vaporizing bottle was first added to the machine in 1930.
- In 1933, dry bobbin type of flow meter was introduced in place of water tight-feed type
- In 1937, Rotameters were displaced with dry bobbin type of flow meters

Besides these, various safety devices like pin-index system, pressure regulators, Triline safety interlock have been introduced. It is now regarded as a good, reliable, useful, safe and most popular machine in every country for the administration of anaesthesia

In this machine, fresh gases are delivered from gas cylinders which are fitted in yoke assembly. High pressure gases pass through the reducing valves to reduce the pressure to about 60 PSI. Pipeline gases are usually supplied at a pressure of 60 PSI. Then these gases pass through metal tubes to rotameter, which contains different flow meters for different gases. The machine incorporates two vaporizing bottles, one for Diethyl Ether and other for Trilene.

Here the Nitrous oxide/Oxygen mixture is directed to get the volatile anaesthetic agent and its concentration may be regulated according to the need of patient. The Gases are allowed to pass through Magill's rebreathing attachment, containing a rubber bag, corrugated rubber tube, expiratory valve and face mask to the patient.

Thus, the anaesthesia machine essentially incorporates a supply of compressed gases, some means to measure the flow of gases and some device for delivery of gases and anaesthetic agents to patient. The components of Boyle's machine are cylinders, cylinder valves, pin index system, (for safe use of the cylinders), pipe line system, pressure gauze, pressure regulators, flow meters, back bar, bag mount, rebreathing bag, corrugated tube and expiratory valve, etc.

CYLINDERS

Boyle's machine is equipped with two Oxygen and two Nitrous oxide cylinders. Modern cylinders are usually made of molybdenum steel to with stand high pressure.

Alloy containing molybdenum (0.15-0.25%) and chromium (0.8 to 1.1%) is used to minimize weight and wall thickness. Walls of the cylinders should be 5/65 to 1/4 inch thick, uniform through out outer side and older cylinders were usually heavier. The cylinders are either solid down or made from stainless steel tube and never welded at ends. After manufacturing process, the cylinders are kept in a furnace, at a temperature between 860° to 890°C and then carefully removed and cooled at atmospheric temperature

Following heat treatment, it should be dried and cleaned completely but no oil or grease should be used inside or outside of the cylinder. All compressed medical and anaesthetic gases, the specification number is ICC 3A and this marking must be placed properly on each cylinder to indicate that it complies with regulators.

All compressed gas cylinders are constructed according to Inter State Commerce Commission Specifications

Cylinders are constructed entirely of steel that meets certain chemical and physical requirements. the walls have minimum thickness of 3/8 inch. Some cylinders are constructed of a chrome molybdenum alloy, which provides a cylinder approximately 20% lighter in weight

Each cylinder is designed to contain a gas under a specified pressure. This is called as service pressure. In addition to specific tensile strength, a cylinder must possess some elasticity but expansion must be subjected to task by interior hydrostatic pressure at least once in every 5 years and it must be recorded. Incorporated in each valve stem is a safety device which under hazardous circumstances of excessive heat or fire will allow the cylinder to becomes exhausted. The device is a simple plug of soft metal alloy called Wood's steel, it is composed of Bismuth, Lead, Tin, and Cadmium. This plug melts at 200^0 F.

Since any gas in a closed container will increase in pressure with a rising temperature, the possibility exists of dangerous pressures being attained. To prevent its occurrence, regulations have been made for safe filling of the cylinders.

Oxygen is also supplied in H or K cylinders 9 OD x 51 containing 220 - 244 cubic feet of gas. Sizes are designated by letters from A to M and the gas capacity advances

Physical states of compressed gases

Nitrous oxide	- Liquid (below 97.7°F)
Cyclopropane	- Liquid (below 256°F)
Ethylene	- Liquid (below 49.1°F)
Oxygen	- Gas
Carbon di oxide	- Liquid (below 88°F)
Helium	- Gas

Rules for handling the Cylinders

Special care must be taken at all times in handling the cylinders with compressed gases. This is important in regard to safety

1. Never permit oil, grease or other readily combustible substances to come in contact with cylinders, valves, regulators, gauzes, hoses and fittings
2. Never lubricate the valves, regulators or fittings
3. Do not handle cylinders with oily hands or gloves
4. Connections to piping, regulators should be tight to prevent leaking
5. Never use an open flame to detect gas leaks. Use soapy water
6. Prevent sparks and flames in vicinity of cylinders
7. Never interchange the regulators with each other
8. Fully open the valve when the cylinders is in use
9. Never attempt to mix the gases in cylinders
10. Cylinder label should be carefully and closely checked and then only remove the wrapping
11. Do not remove the markings and tag
12. No part of the cylinder containing a compressed gas should be subjected to temperature above 1250 F
13. Never attempt with the safety relief valves or cylinders
14. Never attempt to repair or alter the cylinders by your self, this should be done only in presence of service engineer
15. Never use the labelled cylinder for any other purpose other than specified pharmacological use of that gas in that cylinder
16. Never store the cylinders near electric supply
17. Cylinder valves should be closed at all times except when the gas cylinder is in use
18. Cylinders should be repaired and reprinted by suppliers
19. Compressed gases should be handled by experienced and officially trained persons

Colour Code of Cylinders

A colour code to aid in identification of gas cylinders was adopted in 1949 by The Medical Gas Industry. The codes recommend that anaesthetic gas cylinders approximately 4.5' in diameter and 26' length and smaller for use in anaesthesia machine :

- Oxygen - Green, White (international code 1 black body with white shoulder)
- Nitrous oxide - Light blue
- Cyclopropane - Orange
- Carbon dioxide - Gray

Hydraulic test or Pressure test

The test is usually done by water jacket method. Water proof pressure applied inside is 236.2 kg/cm^2 then pressure inside a full cylinder is

- Oxygen - 2000 lbs/inch2
- Nitrous oxide - 750 lbs/inch2
- Carbon di oxide - 720 lbs/inch2
- Air - 2000 lbs/inch2

PIN INDEX SYSTEM

The cylinders are locked to Boyle's machine in metal yoke with two pins and corresponding filling holes on the cylinder head. Each particular cylinder has a fixed pin code. Unless the correct valve is attached, the pins and holes will not coincide and thus it is practically impossible to fit any cylinder to wrong yokes

The positions of holes over the cylinder valve are predetermined. A line is drawn through the center of valve outlet at an angle of 30° to right of valve face. The central point of position 1 passes through it. The central point of position or other positions are located at intervals of 12°. The diameter of valve is 7 mm ± 0.2 mm. the distance between the center of valve outlet and the center of pinhole is 14.3 mm and diameter of pinhole is 4.8 ± mm

There are in all total 6 pins positions on the yoke and 6 holes in cylinder valve. Thus it gives 10 different combinations using 2 hole positions in the cylinder valve and corresponding pin positions on yokes. Following pin positions are accepted

- For oxygen   2 & 5
- For Nitrous oxide   3 & 5
- For cyclopropane   3 & 6
- For carbon di oxide   1 & 6
- For air   1 & 5

The pin index safety system, introduced in 1952. It is an additional and positive safe guard and does not replace any of existing means of preventing wrong connections or for identifying medical gas cylinders

FLOW METERS

A flow meter is a device for measuring quantities of gas while in motion. The working principle denotes that it depends on the laws of flow of fluids in tubes. These are two types :

- Variable orifice meter
- Constant orifice meter

These are designed as wet or dry meters

1. Variable Orifice Meter

The most popular class of flow meters in anaesthesia is variable orifice meters and also known as the Thorpe tube or dry float flow meter. In these flow meters there is a constant pressure difference across an orifice, the size of orifice varies with the flow rate of gas. With a constant pressure difference, the flow rate is proportional to the area of orifice. The basic construction of these meters consists of a glass tube where bore lumen increases from below (inlet) upwards (outlet) and a metering float which moves up and down in tube. The float is so sized that it essentially occludes the lower small inlet port. Since the tube is tapered it follows that as this float is forced upwards by a stream of gas orifice i.e. the space above the float increases

There are two types of constrictions or passage ways. First, the tubular constriction where the diameter of passage way is smaller than the length of constriction. Second, the orifice true one, where the diameter is greater than the length of constriction. Thus in lower positions of most of flow tubes the diameter of channel is essentially of a tubular nature. the viscosity of gas then plays the main role in determining the rate of flow of gas

This is there when small volumes are flowing. Where the constriction is a true orifice, the density of gas plays the dominant role in determining rate of flow. In this instance, the volume of flow of gas is inversely proportional to square root of the gas density

The performance of variable orifice meter is influenced by the changes in density of gas being measured. Temperature also affects the performance, a decrease in temperature may lower the volume flow but the actual mass flow of gas will be greater

Heid-brink meter

This consists of conical metal tube containing a light rod, whose top projects into a calibrated tube. The metal tube does not taper uniformly but widens rapidly in the upper part. Hence, wide range of readings is possible but the accuracy is limited

Rotameter

This consists of a bobbin float, which moves up and down, in a uniformly tapered glass tube. Since there is a variable orifice and flow rates are directly proportional to the area of orifice, These results a linear scale with equal spacing for equal increments of flow

Connell meter

This meter consists of a float of two balls contained in a tapered glass tube mounted on an inclined plane. A stream of gas enters beneath the balls and forces them up. Since the topper of tube measures small flow rates and the upper part, large volumes of flow.

Flow meter measures the flow rate of gas when it passes through it. A flow of accurate concentrations of anaesthetic gases can be adjusted by applying a steady pressure to individual needle valves.

Pin or needle valve consists of a fine pin with a tapered end which fits a ground metal seal. To increase the gas flow, the valve is turned in an anti-clockwise direction.

The flow meter is an accurately tapered glass tube with a light weight bobbin, spinning in gas flow. The bore of tube is tapered, so that the gap in tube wall and bobbin is variable. Gas enters the bottom of flow meter tube and emerges at the top.

The bobbin is lifted by the gas until upward pressure caused by the gas escaping around bobbin and weight of the bobbin rises in tube, greater the gas flows around it. This corresponds to the gas pressure difference below and above the bobbin, which is always constant.

At high flows there is laminar gas flows around it. This corresponds to the gas pressure difference below and above the bobbin, which is always constant.

At high flow rates of gas, the flow is turbulent but at low flows there is laminar gas flow. At high flow rates the clearance is shorter and wider and behaves as an orifice.

The bobbin is made of aluminum and has flutes cut into it. When gas flows with the help of flutes the bobbin spins. Spinning must be well away from the walls of tubes to avoid the errors of friction. Spinning prevents fluctuations of gas flows and reduces the wear and tear.

A white dot is marked on the wall of bobbin. It provides clear indication that the bobbin is rotating freely. Gas flow is read from the flat top of bobbin. Bobbin should be made antistatic to prevent sticking to the wall of flow meter due to static electricity. Static electricity may alter the flow meter output and even cause anaesthetic explosion.

The flow meters are not interring changeable, as the gases in common use have no contact relationship between their density and viscosity.

The flow meter unit is fitted to Boyle's apparatus, incorporates rotating bobbin flow meter tubes for four different gases.

Oxygen graduated in 100 ml / min, 1000 ml / min to 2000 ml / min.

Nitrous oxide graduated 1 lit divisions upto 10 lit/min. Four tubes are contained within a chromium platted metal casing and are protected from dust and damage by a plastic window.

Each flow meter knob is colour coded for gas as white for oxygen, blue for Nitrous oxide. Flow meter mal-function may include leaks and obstruction.

In accurate reading may occur due to bobbin stuck, distorted and damaged bobbin, improper alignment of wrong gas for flow meter.

Flow meters should be set in vertical position. Inclined position gives incorrect reading by causing friction on the wall by bobbin, by making the annulus, asymmetrical and also causing resistance on gas flow.

Flow meters can give inaccurate readings by back pressure and extreme temperatures.

BOYLES' MAJOR ANAESTHESIA MACHINE

Boyle's major is basically and structurally similar to Boyles' F model but it is some what bigger in size.

- It provides provision for 3 Oxygen, 2 Nitrous oxide and 1 Carbob dioxide/Cyclopropane cylinder and provision of 2 central oxygen pipeline supply. All the cylinders are fitted with appropriate preset regulators.
- It has one large table top, one instrument trolley, one detachable drawer at base.
- The swivel outlet lies at the right front corner of the apparatus and the other end there is provision for connecting circle absorber.
- The swivel outlet has a spiring loaded emergency oxygen control. A flexible or detachable connection is plugged into the swivel outlet, so the anaesthetic gases mixture is conducted to the fixed outlet on the left front of apparatus.
- Cylinder yokes are pin-indexed to the international standards and are colour coded. Non-interchanble threaded inlet

connections are provided to connect pipeline outlets directly to the apparatus.

• Rotating bobbin flow meters used in the machine have 230 mm caliberated tubes, each tube mounted in an individual assembly with its own flow control needle valves. The needle valve control knobs are colour coded for each gas (White for Oxygen, Blue for Nitrous oxide and black or gray for Carbon dioxide or cyclopropane).

• A detachable luminous back plate is there behind the flow meters so that in dark flow meters and bobbin movements due to flow of gases can be identified.

• A pressure gauge is fitted to each of the yokes and each pipeline inlet of the apparatus.

• Vaporizers for Ether and Trichloroethylene can be attached on back bar with vaporizer circuit control valve.

• There is one combined non-return or blow-off valve at right top to vent the excess of gases at pressure more than 100 cm of water. This prevents entry of gases from the breathing circuit entering back into vaporizer.

• There is arrangement for closed circuit.

Other Anaesthesia machines

1. Boyles' mark-III anaesthesia machine
2. King's portable anaesthesia machine
3. Boyles' portable anaesthesia machine
4. Medisys – supreme anaesthesia machine
5. MRI anaesthesia machine

12

Endotracheal Equipments

LARYNGOSCOPE

Laryngoscope is used to visualize the larynx and adjacent structures, most commonly for the purpose of insertion of endotracheal tube into tracheal tree. These may be from simple rigid blade laryngoscope to complex fibre-optic laryngoscope

RIGID LARYNGOSCOPE

Most laryngoscopes in use today, consists of a handle and one detachable blade. The light source is energized when the blade and handle are locked in working position.

Handle

- The handle provides power supply for light
- It is having disposable dry battery cells
- Fibre-optic self illuminated laryngoscopes has remote light source
- Most of the handles are designed to accept either fibre-optic, illuminated or lamp in bulb blades
- Hook on (hinged folding) connection between handle and blade is most commonly used

- The handle is placed or fitted with a hinge pin that fits a slot on the base of blade. This allows quick and easy attachment and detachment
- Handles are designed to accept blades that have a light bulb with a metallic contact which completes the electrical circuit, when handle and blades are in working position
- When the handle and blade are locked in working position, an activator switch is depressed. This provides a connection between bulb and battery. Illumination is better with lamp in blade than fibre-optic system, use of mains power may improve the brightness
- Handles are available in several sizes. Short handles may be advantageous for patients in whom chest or breasts contacts the handle during use, when cricoid pressure is being applied or when the patient is in body cast
- Most of handles form a right angle with the blade, when ready for use, the angle may be acute or obtuse
- Handle has serrations or roughness to have firm grip of handle
- Standard handle accepts two size 'C' 1.5 volts batteries.
- Penlight handle – it has advantage of intubating paediatric patient and accepts two size AA 1.5 volts batteries.
- Stubby blade – designed to accommodate the difficult on a short neck, barrel chest, large blossomed patient, where the distance between the mouth and the chest prohibits the use of standard length blade. It accepts two size AA 1.5 volts batteries.

Blade

- The blade is rigid component that is inserted into the mouth
- The blades are numbered with number increasing with size
- Disposable blades are also present and available
- The blade is composed of several parts including the base, heel, tongue, flange, web, tip and light source
- The base is the part, that attaches to the handle. It has a slot for engaging the hinges pin of the handle. The proximal end of base is called heel

- The tongue (spatula) is main shaft. It serves to compress and manipulate the soft tissues (especially tongue) and lower jaw. The long axis of tongue (spatula) may be straight or curved in part or all of its length. Blades are commonly referred to as curved or straight, depending on predominant slope of spatula
- The flange projects off the side of spatula and is connected to it by webs. It serves to guide instrumentation and deflect the tissues out of the line of vision. The flange determine the cross sectional shape of blade. The vertical height of cross sectional shape of blade is some times referred to as the step.
- The tip (beak) contacts either with epiglottis or vallecula and directly or indirectly elevates the epiglottis. It is usually blunt and thickened to decrease the chances of trauma
- The blade has a lamp (bulb) or a fibre-optic handle, that transmits light from the source in handle
- The bulb screws into a socket, which is located near the tip. On some blade, it is at base. When the blade is snapped into the place, electrical contact with batteries in the handle is made. The socket is subjected to soiling by fluids that can affect the electrical contacts causing the light to fail.
- Use of laryngoscope presents little or no difficulty to the experienced operator and skill is of more importance than the type of blade employed

VARIOUS TYPES OF BLADES

1. McIntosh blade

It is one of the most popular blade. Tongue (spatula) has a smooth, gentle curve that extends upto the tip. There is a flange at the left, to push the spatula out of the way. In cross section, the spatula, web & flange form a inverse Z. The number 4 blade may be more useful than number 3 in normal & healthy adults because the smallest portion of the blade will often lie out of vision of mouth, during intubation.

Size 00	Premature	70 mm
Size 0	Neonatal	80 mm

Size 1	Infant	92 mm
Size 2	Child	100 mm
Size 3	Adult	130 mm
Size 4	Large adult	155 mm
Size 5	Extra large	178 mm

2. Left handed MacIntosh blade

Left handed MacIntosh blade has the flange on the opposite from usual McIntosh blade. This blade may be useful for left handed persons (anaesthesits), Intubating in the right lateral position and positioning a tracheal tube directly from the left side of mouth. Size 3 for adults 130 mm.

3. Miller blade

- It is one of the most popular blade
- The spatula is straight with slight upward curve near tip
- In cross section, the flange, web and spatula form C with the tip flattened
- The lamp socket is on spatula, where as other versions have it on the web

Size 00	Premature	57 mm
Size 0	Neonatal	75 mm
Size 0.5	Small infant	88 mm
Size 1	Infant	102 mm

- Only Mcintosh blades of sizes 0, 1, 2, 3 and 4 and Miller blades 0 and 1 are available in satin finish there by eliminating reflection and glare.

TRUPTI BLADES - With flexible Articulating Tip

Ideally suited for use in patients where there is anticipated difficult intubation. Trupti blade simplifies the elevation of the epiglottis and exposure of the larynx, thereby reducing the force required for laryngoscopy.

Applications include the situations where forward displacement of the larynx, forward or prominent upper teeth (buck teeth), large tongue, backward displacement of tongue, decreased neck movements, cervical spine injuries, decreased mouth opening and recessive mandible.

Silent features are :

- Size 3 – adult – 130 mm
- Size 4 – Large adult – 155 mm
- There is no need for separate handle, it can fit to hook – on type of handle
- Articulating tip provides precise control to elevate the epiglottis
- Channel to visualize the epiglottis and facilitate the insertion of an endotracheal tube
- Unobstructed view
- Unique anti-seize spring action
- Optimal smooth action
- Precision made for ruggedness and high quality
- Full stainless steel construction
- Conventional lamp type
- Fits on all hook-on handles
- Economical
- Paediatric version is not available

Fibre – optic Laryngoscope blade

- Hook-on handle used with convential blades can be used with Fibrolite blades. There is no need to have special handle.
- No trauma causing hot bulb
- No possibility of loose bulb entering oral airway
- Cool high power light
- No electrical wires in the blades
- No flickering
- There is steady, bright and focused beam.

- These are of standard McIntosh blades.
- Over 3000 fibers bundled together ensures steady, bright and focused beam.
- It is available in Matt finish at no extra cost.
- These are manufactured in India so easily available with all spare parts and service facility.

COMPLICATIONS OF LARYNGOSCOPY

1. Dental injury

- Damage to teeth, gums, dental prosthesis
- Foreign body dislodgment into the tracheo - bronchial tree
- Bleeding from surrounding area and aspiration
- Teeth or prosthetic device may be clipped, broken, loosened or avulsed
- Upper incisors are commonly involved in this problem
- Protruded teeth may cause difficulty in laryngoscopy and intubation. It will enhance the problem, when other associated criteria for causing difficulty in intubation are present
- The tooth protector may prevent dental damage
- The placement of adhesive tapes on flange may minimize the problem to some extent.

2. Damage to soft tissues and nerves

The injuries may cause abrasion, hematoma, laceration of lips, tongue, palate, pharynx, hypopharynx, larynx and oesophagus. Rolling of lip between teeth and blade. Laryngeal nerve may be injured

3. Injury to cervical cord

Aggressive positioning of the head during intubation especially extension of head or neck, may cause damage in unstable cervical spine as in malformation, fractures or dislocation or tumour

4. Circulatory system changes

- Laryngoscopy may result in significant haemodynamic changes. These changes varies with the type of blade used
- Curved blade laryngoscope, which rest at the superior portion of epiglottis and results in sympathetic stimulation as resultant tachycardia and hypertension
- Straight blade laryngoscopy in which epiglottis is taken up into blade, it stimulates parasympathetic system and results in bradycardia and hypotension
- If laryngoscopy is performed in light plane of anaesthesia it results in either sympathetic or parasympathetic stimulation causing either tachycardia or bradycardia and hypertension or hypotension or both
- It may result in dangerous dysarrhythmia which may be many times more dangerous in patients who are having already severe cardiovascular disorders like severe hypertension, shock due to any reasons, heart block, coronary artery disease, myocardial ischemia or infarction, cardiac failure due to any cause, fixed cardiac output states, etc
- Swallowing or aspiration of foreign body
- It may bulb of laryngoscope or teeth

5. Shock or burn

- If laryngoscope light is left on, contacts with patient's skin and burn may result
- Malpositioning of blade on handle can produce a short circuit, which leads to heating of handle and can cause shock or burn. Which leads to heating of handle and can cause shock or burn

6. Laryngoscope malfunction

- Inability to fix the blade on handle
- Failure of light source even though battery cells are not exhausted

- Due to loss of serrations on the handle due to prolonged use and it may become slippery
- Crust formation at handle end and blade end so no chemical reaction at the site of contact of handle and blade.
- The tracheal tubes (endotracheal tube, intra-tracheal tube and catheter) is inserted into trachea and is used to conduct anaesthesia gases and anaesthetic vapors, to pass to and fro into lungs

ENDTRACHEAL TUBES

Materials of constructions

The material from which a tracheal tube is manufactured should have the following characteristics

1. It should have low cost
2. These should have lack of tissue toxicity
3. These should be as far as transparent
4. These should have ease of sterilization and these should have long durability with repeated sterilization
5. These should be non-inflammable
6. The tube should have a smooth, non-wetable surface inside and outside to prevent built up of secretions, it allows easy passage of a suction catheter or bronchoscope and prevent trauma.
7. It should have sufficient sturdiness to maintain its shape during insertion and prevent occlusion by torsion, kinking and compression by the cuff or external pressure
8. It should have sufficient strength to allow thin wall construction
9. These should have non-reactivity with lubricants and the agents used in anaesthesia

No substance with all these criteria has been found.

For many years, tracheal tubes were made from rubber. These tubes can be cleaned, sterilized and can be used multiple times. These are not transparent, harden and become sticky after prolonged use. These have poor resistance to kinking, become clogged by incepted secretions more easily than the plastic tubes and do not soften at body temperature. Latex allergy is another possible problem

At present, Poly-vinyl chloride (PVC) is the substance most widely used in disposable tracheal tubes. It is relatively in expensive and compatible with the tissues. These tubes have fewer tendencies to kinking than rubber tubes. These are stiff enough for endotracheal intubation at room temperature but soften at body temperature so that These tend to confirm to the anatomy of patients upper airway, There by reducing the pressure at the points of contact

Poly-vinyl chloride tube may be refrigerated to make it more firm for intubation or warmed prior to use to facilitate the placement over a fibroscope. These have a smooth surface that facilitates the passage of a suction catheter or bronchoscope. Their transparency permits the observation of tidal movements of the respiratory moisture as well as objects or materials in side lumen

Silicone is used in the manufacturing of some of tubes. It is more expensive than PVC. It can be sterilized or reused. Some materials used in the manufacture of tracheal tubes in the past have shown evidence of tissue toxicity.

- Low volume - High pressure cuff
- High volume/low pressure cuff
- Inflation system
- Inflation lumen

The inflation lumen which connects the inflation tube to the cuff is located within wall of tracheal tube. It should not encroach on the lumen of tube and recommends that, it should not bulge outward

External inflation tube

The external inflation tube (cuff tube, pilot tube, pilot balloon line, inflating tube, tail) is external to the tube. The external diameter should not exceed 2.5 mm, and it is attached to the tube at a small angle. The standard red rubber tube also specifies that the distance from tube tip to the tube is attachment and requires that the tube extend at least 3 cm beyond the machine end of tube before pilot balloon inflation valve is incorporated

The inflation tube can become obstructed by kinking or by crushing from a clamp

On spiral embedded tubes, the inflating tube may connect to inflation lumen above the first spiral ring. If the connector is inserted into the tube far enough to contact first spiral, it may cause the inflation tube to blockage

Pilot balloon

The pilot balloon (bulb, external reservoir, external balloon) may be located near the mid point of the inflating tube or adjacent to the inflation valve. Its function is to give an indication of the inflation or deflation of cuff

Inflation valve

The external inflation tube with either fitted to an inflation valve, with an inlet that will fix with a male latex syringe tip or have female end capable of occupying a standard luer tip syringe. Portex (PVC) tubes has one way inflation valve and rubber tubes have cap over inflation valve and these are two way

ENDOTRACHEAL CONNECTIONS

- Endotracheal connections are generally curved metal tubes and plastic varieties are also available
- One end of connection connects with the endotracheal tube and other end connects to the catheter mount
- The addition of the connectors to an endotracheal tube increases the resistance. Curved connections produce more resistance than straight variety of connecting.
- The gas flow becomes more turbulent & less laminar in right angled connections than in curved connections
- A connection has two ends, one is the patient end and the other is machine end

- Some connections also provide an opening for the suction. This opening is always kept closed by rubber or metal cap except at the time of suctioning
- The end which connects to tube is distal or patient end and its size denotes the internal diameter in mm. Various sizes are available, usually with the increments of 0.5 mm up to 3 mm and then with increment of 1 mm above 3 mm size
- The correct size of connection should be chosen so as to get the wide lumen of endotracheal tube and connection has snuggly fitting
- The end which connects with breathing system is known as proximal or machine end and it has a standard 15 mm male fitting (outside diameter)
- The connected ends should be leak proof, minimum reduction of lumen and never to be dislodged or disconnected easily
- The endotracheal connections may increase the mechanical dead space and it may be significantly excessive for neonates or infants
- Metal endotracheal connections may be autoclaved
- 15 mm plastic disposable connections of Portex are also available

Magill's Metal Connections

Row Bothum connections

Cobb's and Magill's Suction Union

Noseworthy Portex Connections

INDICATIONS OF ENDOTRACHEAL INTUBATION

Group I

The intubation is mandatory - patient's life depends on the use of endotracheal tube. No patient in this group should be operated under general anaesthesia, without endotracheal intubation

- Intra-cranial operations
- Intra-thoracic operations
- Operations, which are performed in prone position

- Very major operative procedures
- Intestinal obstructions or the patient with full stomach
- Major head and neck surgery
- Intra-oral surgery like tonsillectomy and operations on tongue
- Major intra-abdominal surgery

Group II

- Endotracheal intubation is preferable, intubation affords greater safety or superior operating conditions or field
- Minor head neck surgery
- Minor thoracic surgery
- Minor intra-abdominal surgery
- Operative positions compromising body physiology like lateral position or kidney position

Group III

- Intubation optional advantages and disadvantages are balanced
- Operations on extremities
- Minor superficial surgery on the body

Group IV

- Intubation is not necessary
- Minor surgery procedure, like incision and drainage of abscess dressings, fracture reductions, anal dilatation etc

Other Indications of Endotracheal intubation

1. Cardio-pulmonary resuscitation
2. Aspiration pneumonitis
3. Terminal stages of illness
4. Respiratory paralysis due to any cause in intensive care unit
5. Eletro-convulsive therapy
6. Poisoning due to any agents

7. Neuro-muscular paralysis central or peripheral due to any cause
8. Resuscitation of new born
9. Drowning, suffocation, carbon monoxide poisoning
10. Head injury or facio-maxillary injuries as an air way
11. Postoperatively, when the patient is not completely out of anaesthesia effects or any post operative complication
12. As a treatment part in high or total spinal anaesthesia

Advantages of Endotracheal intubation

1. It provides a free unobstructed airway
2. There is decrease in respiratory effort
3. It provides the control of airway
4. There is increase in respiratory relaxation
5. It facilitates the prevention of pulmonary aspiration
6. Helpful for control of the ventilation
7. One can provide assisted ventilation
8. It facilitates cardiopulmonary resuscitation
9. One can keep the patient, anaesthesists and the machine away from the surgical field
10. It diminishes the anatomical as well as the physiological dead space in patient

Disadvantages

1. For successful endotracheal intubation, it requires the technical skill of anaesthetists
2. The technique of endotracheal intubation requires thorough knowledge of anatomy and physiology of the respiratory tract and the physiology of respiration
3. For endotracheal intubation deeper planes of anaesthesia are required
4. Some times it requires prolonged time to perform intubation
5. There are chances of kinking of tube and resulting obstruction

6. There are chances of leak from the side of tube as small size of tube has to be passed and due to that, there is wastage of anaesthesia gases and chances of pollution
7. During the act of intubation, there are chances of various types of arrhythmias
8. Due to tedious act of intubation, there are chances of trauma to upper respiratory tract
9. In the light planes of anaesthesia, it may provoke cough, breath holding and some times bronchospasm

Perioperative complications of tracheal tubes

1. **Trauma :**
   - The intubation is often associated with trauma to the structures of upper and lower airway. 80% of the patients may have occult or visible blood after extubation
   - The trauma is often associated with the use of excessive force or repeated attempts of intubation
   - It varies with the skill of anaesthesists,the difficulty during act of intubation and amount of muscle relaxation. The damage may be enhanced if a stylet protrudes the end of tube or through Murphys' eye
   - Mucosa can be torned when a metal or foil wrapped tube is used
   - The plastic tubes become stiffer when kept in cold atmosphere and may increase the chances of trauma while on insertion
   - Trauma to lips, tongue, teeth, nose, pharynx, trachea and or bronchus may occur. These injuries are from simple abrasion to severe laceration and perforation have been reported
   - Temporo-mandibular joint dislocation have been reported
   - During nasal intubation, trauma may occur as avulsion, tear, perforation of nasal septum, adenoid perforation and severe bleeding

- Trauma may occur during extubation to vocal cords, trachea and valeculi
- To avoid perioperative trauma gentle pressure and patient movements should well guided. Stylet should be flexible and never extend beyond bevel or Murphy eye
- Use of vasoconstrictors, warming of tube, sequential dilatation will reduce the chances of trauma during nasal intubation
- Lubrication of tube before insertion will also reduce the chances of trauma

2. **Failure to achieve satisfactory sealing :**
   - A leaking cuff or tube make the maintenance of adequate ventilation difficult, failure to protect against aspiration and oral surgery difficult to perform
   - The connector may also produce leak

3. **Oesophageal intubation :** It can be avoided or recognized by
   - Direct visualization
   - By feel of reservoir bag
   - Chest wall movements on ventilation will be absent
   - On auscultation there will not be any breath sounds. There will be gurgling sounds over stomach area on auscultation
   - There will be sounds or air around tube
   - There will be epigastric distension after some time
   - There will not be condensation of moisture inside of tube, which will be evident with PVC tube
   - There will be gastric contents in side tube
   - Due to oesophageal intubation, there will be failure of oxygenation
   - Chest X-ray will confirm oesophageal intubation
   - There will not be palpable substernal notch
   - Use of fibroscope will confirm the oesophageal intubation
   - One may confirm by tactile method, that feel of bag will be different and there will not be bag movements of respiratory cycle i.e. during inspiration and expiration

- The bronchial placement lead to atelectasis of non-ventilated lung and decreased oxygenation. The lung that is ventilated may become hyper inflated leading to barotrauma and hypoxia
- It is found more frequently during emergency, paediatric patients and in female patients
- Usually right sided bronchial intubation is most common
  It is detected by :
  - Bilateral auscultation for air entry
  - Visualization of symmetrical movements of chest expansion
  - X-ray chest for detection
  - The position of tube at lips and nostrils, it is less important
  - By noting the guide marks on tracheal tube which shows that less markings are remaining outside
  - It can be confirmed by auscultation of breath sounds which are usually absent or less on opposite side
  - Estimation of expired carbon dioxide tension which is less in bronchial intubation
  - It can be confirmed by pulse oximetry which shows less oxygen saturation
4. Foreign body aspiration : A tracheal tube may dislodge fragments of tissues from oral cavity, pharynx or larynx, adenoids, teeth, blood, etc
5. There are chances of leak even though the tube is inside
6. Rarely there might be airway perforation
7. There might be complication related to Murphy eye
8. Laser radiation induced tracheal tube fires
9. There might be cautery induced fires
10. Aspiration of stomach contents: It is possible with
    Low pressure cuffs
    When patient is on spontaneous ventilation
    When there is accumulation of fluid above the cuff

In head up position

When non-cuffed tube pharyngeal packing is used

11. There are chances of Accidental extubation

12. Systemic bacteremia, when the patient is already having active infection prior to intubation, URI, chest infection, etc

13. Some times, there might be difficulty in extubation which is due to non deflation of cuff, partial deflation and wrinkling of cuff

14. Postoperative sore throat when preoperative URI is present

15. Post operative hoarseness of voice chances are there, when large size tube is forcefully passed, over inflation of cuff, when the cuff has rested on vocal cords, prolonged intubation and vocal cord palsy

16. There are chances of various nerve injuries like trigeminal, lingual, buckle and glossopharngeal nerves

17. In the post operative period, there are chances of upper airway oedema

18. There might be vocal cord dysfunction postoperatively

19. There are chances of laceration of trachea and larynx during the act of intubation

20. After prolonged intubation, there are chances of development of granuloma of vocal cords

21. There are chances of laryngo-tracheal membrane formation

22. There might be formation of glottic and sub-glottic granulation

23. During nasal intubation, there are chances of damage to nose

24. Very rarely, there are chances of tracheal stenosis postoperatively on prolonged intubation

25. Some times, the patients may develop latex allergy

26. There are every chances of endotracheal tube obstruction due to various reasons as - Biting of tube, kinking, foreign material inside lumen of tube, bevel touching against tracheal wall, herniation of cuff, external compression, defective connectors, etc.

COMPLICATIONS OF ENDOTRACHEAL INTUBATION

Mishaps related to equipments

- Kinking or collapse
- Respiratory obstruction due to any cause
- When the internal diameter of tube is too small, then it may cause resistance to ventilation
- When the tube is too long, then it will increase the dead space
- The layer's of latex may peel off forming a flap and obstruction

Problems due to stylet

- Plastic stylet may break, free in trachea or bronchus
- Too long stylet may lacerate larynx or trachea

Problems due to Laryngoscope

- Bulb may go off or dimmed
- Bulb may drop down and act as foreign body

Problems of cuff

- The pressure of cuff may obstruct ciliary functions
- Cuff may overlap the end of tube, causing obstruction
- Cuff may have wrinkling or may collapse resulting in difficulty in extubation many times

Problems due to use of lubricants

- Oil of lubricant may cause lipoid pneumonia
- Water may cause oedema
- Water soluble jellies may dry & cause obstruction
- Xylocaine jelly is less harmful
- Some times Xylocaine jelly may prose the problem of aspiration or obtund cough reflex due to local anaesthetic action. It may cause difficulty in coughing post operatively

Problems due to packs

- Threads of gauze may come in airway
- Pack may be inadvertently left inside throat
- Pressure of pack may be on larynx causing oedema

Mishaps of intubation

1. Trauma

- Trauma to lips, teeth, gums and denture
- Stretching of pharyngeal muscles causing subluxation of jaw
- Trauma to larynx, pharynx and epiglottis
- Nasal bleeding, trauma to adenoids
- Some times it may cause mediastinal emphysema, mediastinitis

2. Reflex disturbances

- Various cardiac arrhythmias, there might be bradycardia due to vagal stimulation and tachycardia due to sympathetic stimulation
- Vasovagal reflex stimulation due to non-atropinization or parasympathetic stimulatory action
- There might be occurrence of apnea, breath-holding, coughing or bucking after intubation, when intubation is carried out in light planes of anaesthesia

3. Problems due to Positioning

- If too far inserted inside then, there will right bronchial intubation, left lung will not be ventilated and chances of atelectasis
- There are chances of obstruction due to touching of bevel against the tracheal wall
- The cuff may be caught in between two cords and there by chances of injury to cords and hoarseness of voice postoperatively

4. Problems due to foreign body

- If caught between the cords, then chances of oedema of cords and also erythematic and difficulty in respiration postoperatively
- If the cuff is inflated more than the pressure of cuff wall, which presses the tracheal mucosa anteriorly / posteriorly and there are chances of development of necrosis of tracheal wall

MAGILL'S ENDOTRACHEAL TUBES

- These are made of India rubber, so red in colour
- These have anti-static property due to rubber and the humidification during expired air
- These are available in all sizes, starting from No. 2 to No. 11 in variants of 0.5 mm according to the internal diameter of tube
- The thickness of tube is constant through out the length from tracheal end to machine end
- Tracheal end has got a bevel. The angle of bevel is angle formed by the tip of bevel to body of tube
- According to the angle of bevel, these can be useful for nasal or oral intubation. In nasal tube the angle of bevel is 30^0 and in oral angle is 45^0.
- The shaft of tube has got radius of curvature. It is acute in the nasal tubes and obtuse in oral tubes
- The radius of curvature is more in nasal tubes 20 cms and less in oral tubes 14 cm
- Length of tubes differs from the size of tube

Differences between Oral / Nasal Endotracheal tubes

- Radius of curvature is more in nasal tube verses oral tube,
- Nasal tubes has sharper curve than oral tubes
- Radius of curvature in oral tube is 14 cm
- Radius of curvature in nasal tubes is 20 cm
- Angle of bevel in nasal tube is 30°.

- Angle of bevel in oral tube is 45°.
- Size of tube : $\dfrac{\text{Age in years}}{2} + 28$
- Length of tube : $\dfrac{\text{Age in years}}{2} + 12$

In adults anatomical measurements useful are :
Mean distance from lips to carina
> Male is 28.5 cm, female is 25.2 cm

Mean distance from base of nose to carina
> Male is 31cm and in females is 28.4 cm

The distance from lips to vocal cords
> Male is 12-16 cm, in females is 10-14 cm

Mean length of trachea (vocal cords to carina)
> Male is 12-14 cm, in female is 10-14 cm

In adults, any tube over 24 cm in length is suitable and can be inserted through vocal cords for a distance of 4-7 cm is desirable

Magill's Plane Endotracheal tube

- It is usually passed nasally or sometimes orally in difficulty
- All times, It is made of India rubber
- It comes in size from 2 mm to 10 mm according to the internal diameter in the variants of 0.5 mm
- It can be oral / nasal or only nasal according to the angle of bevel and radius of curvature
- It is preferably passed nasally and in difficulty or in emergency passed orally
- When the plane tube is passed orally, then it poses the problem of leaking and silent aspiration
- During nasal intubation, it should be first well lubricated and then passed from one of nostril
- To pass a tube by nasal route, it is more easy than orally route in the experienced hands

- Some times nasal intubation does not require laryngoscopy or direct visualization of cords
- Many times nasal intubation requires aid of Magills' forceps, to facilitate intubation when the tube is passed beyond oropharynx
- Nasal intubation requires patency of the nostrils as prime importance without which, it should not be performed

Pre-requisites of Nasal intubation

- Plane endotracheal rubber tube of desirable size and of one less number than oral size tube
- Patency of both nostrils, minimum one nostril
- Bleeding and clotting time estimation
- Magill's forceps
- Throat packing or roll gauze

Indications of Nasal intubation

1. For oral surgery, it is mandatory
   Left lip and cleft palate surgery
   Surgery on tongue i.e. glossectomy, cyst removal, ranula
   Dental surgery
   Intra dental wiring for fracture maxilla or mandible
   Removal of AC polyp
   Maxillectomy or mandibulectomy
   Tonsillectomy
   Intra oral surgery for cheek operations
2. Posterior cranial fossa surgery in lateral position
3. Operations on nape of neck
4. It can be used as airway by nasal route, when oral airway is not tolerated in semiconscious patient or when the pharyngeal or laryngeal reflexes are active
5. In emergency for resuscitation of patient
6. In anticipated difficult intubation by oral route

7. When cuff oral tubes are not available
8. Cuff tubes are some what costly and in practice, when every body can not afford

Contraindications

1. Suspected difficult endotracheal intubation
2. Deviated nasal septum
3. In patients with upper respiratory tract infection
4. Atrophic rhinitis
5. In cases with nasal polyp (*AC polyp*, adenoids, fracture of nasal bone)
6. Retrophyaryngeal abscess
7. Bleeding disorders of any kind
8. When adequate size nasal tube is not available, too small tube produces leak and too large tube can not be passed, it will cause trauma and profuse bleeding
9. When the force is required or cannot be passed easily
10. When only cuff tube is available
11. Smooth induction and intubation is desirable as in occular surgery

MAGILL'S CUFF ENDOTRACHEAL TUBE

- It is made of India red rubber hence red in colour
- It is usually made for oral intubation only but can be passed nasally on rare occasions
- It comes in sizes from 6 mm onwards upto 11 mm in the variants of 0.5 mm but from 2 mm onwards are also available
- Small size cuff tubes from 2–6 mm are not usually manufactured and if present, are not used routinely
- The cuff is low volume and high pressure hence prolonged use is not advocated
- The cuff should be inflated with 2 – 3 ml of air which increases the intra cuff pressure upto 20 – 30 cm of water. It should not

be inflated more than 3 ml at one time, as it when inflated increases the intra cuff pressure above 40 cm of water, which hampers tracheal mucosal perfusion pressure

- It should be deflated intermittently to establish the mucosal blood circulation and there are less chances of sore throat or permanent ischemic damage. When angle of bevel is 45^0 and the radius of curvature is 14 cm.
- Oral cuff tube should not be passed nasally as it causes more trauma to nasal mucosa and one has to pass small size tube, when orally large size is not negotiable
- Snuggly fitting tube insertion should not be under taken, as cuff inflation will increase the external pressure on tracheal mucosa with minimum inflation of cuff.

Indications of Double Lumen tubes or Endo-bronchial Intubation

1. Operations on Lung parenchyma
   Lobectomy
   Pneumonectomy
   Broncho-pleural fistula resection
   Lung abscess
   Bronchogenic carcinoma
   Aspiration of bronchial secretions
   Repair of broncho-pleural cutaneous fistula
   Empyema thoracis
   Thickened pleura
   Bronchiectasis aspiration
   Pulmonary aspiration
2. Pulmonary Operations
   Repair of tracheo-oesophageal fistula
   Operation for ca-oesophagus
   Coarctation aorta
   Thymetcomy
   Mediastinal tumours

3. Differential broncho - spirometery perfusion and ventilation of the individual lung is measured, right lung 55% and left lung 45%
4. For bronchography

HAZARDS ASSOCIATED WITH DOUBLE LUMEN TUBES

1. These have difficulty with insertion and positioning
2. There are chances of mal-position of tube
3. Some times there is unsatisfactory lung deflation
4. There might be obstruction to inflation
5. There are chances of gas trapping with this tube
6. Some times there might be failure of lung separation
7. Hypoxemia may be there due to ventilation/perfusion mismatch
8. There might be obstruction to air flow due to :
   Over inflation of bronchial cuff can cause narrowing of lumen
   Bronchial lumen can become twisted and results in partial obstruction
   Carinal hook may obstruct tracheal lumen
9. It may cause trauma as rupture of main stem bronchus, perforation of trachea, dislodgment of bronchial tumors
10. There may be the problems due to tube itself as distortion of tracheal lumen and splitting of tube
11. Surgical complications as carinal hook may be clamped, bronchial cuff rupture, tight stenosis, etc
12. Very rarely circulatory collapse due to compression of great vessels

13

Day Care Surgery

Day care surgery, Ambulatory surgery or out-patient surgery is defined as one in which the procedure is performed on a patient without overnight hospitalization either before or after surgery.

It is practiced since long back everywhere but becoming very popular in developed countries. Paediatric outpatient anaesthesia was first reported by Nicoll in 1903. In western countries the incidence of day stay surgery is about 50%.

Day care surgery offers certain advantages to the patient, medical staff and community.

It reduces the cost of medical care.

It avoids prolonged or un-necessary hospital stay.

Reduces the chances of exposure to hospital acquired infection.

Minimal psychological disturbances particularly in paediatric patients i.e. separation from family and home environment.

Quick disposal of patients as no waiting period for operation,

Inturn it provides enough accommodation for needy indoor patients.

The basic principles of ambulatory surgery were originally applied to healthy children and adults undergoing minor operations.

There is increasing evidence that arbitory limits placed on the type of surgery, age of the patient, duration of operation, preoperative fasting period and selection of perioperative medication may be warranted.

Over last decade, an increasing number of high risk patients have presented for outpatient surgery, making proper selection and evaluation to be important. Still now, the recovery time is too long and incidence of common side effects is high.

Benefits of Ambulatory Surgery

- Patient's preference, especially children and elderly.
- Lack of dependence on availability of hospital beds.
- Greater flexibility in scheduling operations.
- Low incidence of perioperative morbidity and mortality.
- Lower incidence of hospital acquired infection.
- Lower incidence of postoperative respiratory complications.
- Higher volume of patients.
- Shorter surgical waiting list.
- Lower procedural cost.
- Less preoperative testing and postoperative medication.

These factors all contribute to 25–75% reduction in overall cost for most of the operations performed in outpatient setting.

Ambulatory surgical facilities need to be well designed to ensure optimal delivery of surgical services at reduced cost.

The patient volume, type of patients and procedures, organizational structure, radiological and laboratory testing must all be considered during initial planning of new facility. Design of the place, waiting room, pre-anaesthesia room, operating suits and recovery areas in close proximity.

Quality assurance and total quality improvement are necessary to maintain high standards for out patient care and to ensure safety.

Accreditation Association for Ambulatory Health Care (AAAHC) is an independent accreditation organization whose principal activities are the development of standards, the conduct of surveys and conforming the accreditation. ASA also provides the guidelines for conduction.

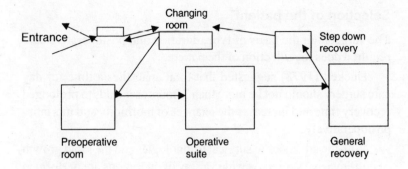

ESSENTIAL COMPONENTS OF AMBULATORY SURGERY

Anaesthesiologists need to be involved in the initial planning and organization of these facilities to ensure safe, efficient and economic patient care.

Patient Selection

Operative procedures suitable for ambulatory surgery :

- Dental – Extraction, restoration, facial fractures
- Skin – Excision of skin lesions, warts, lipoma, lymph nodes, cysts,etc.
- General – Biopsy, endoscopies, excision of benign tumors.
- Gynecology – Cervical dilatation & curettage, hystroscopy, laproscopy, tubal ligation, *vaginal hysterectomy.*
- Ophthalmology – Cataract extraction, chalazion removal, probing, tonometry, foreign body removal.
- Orthopaedic – Closed fracture reduction, arthroscopy, manipulations, nail removal, nailing under image intensifier.
- ENT — Laryngoscopy, myringotomy, polypectomy, tympano-plasty.
- Pain clinic – Chemical sympathectomy, epidural injection, nerve blocks.
- Plastic surgery – Cleft lip repair, skin grafting.
- Urology – Circumcision, cystoscopy, lithotripsy.

Selection of the patient

The surgeon on the basis of type, duration and postoperative care required does the selection of the patient.

Duckett (1978) suggested that total anaesthesia time for day care surgery should not be more than 2 hours as it leads to prolonged recovery time and increases the chances of morbidity and mortality postoperatively.

With the advances in surgical technologies and the rapid growth of non-invasive surgery, a wide variety of operations are performed on the outpatient basis.

Most patients of ambulatory surgery are ASA physical status I and II.

Extremes of ages i.e. less than 6 months and more than 70 years are accepted to require prolong postoperative care so not selected for day care surgery.

The preoperative assessment of outpatients has become increasingly important because patients are presenting for ambulatory surgery with more complex medical conditions. So it is essential to develop a method of screening these patients preoperatively in order to avoid costly delays and last time cancellation.

Computerized interview may efficiently solve the problem.

The patients requiring specific anaesthetic consideration or these with high risk and surgical complications should be identified in preoperative visit.

Thorough patient preparation prior to the day of surgery can prevent un-necessary delays, absences, last time cancellation and inadequate patient management.

Optimal preoperative preparation of outpatients makes ambulatory surgery both safer and more acceptable for patients and hospital staff. The preparation process is aimed at reducing the risk, improving patients outcome and making the surgical experience pleasant for the patient and family members.

Quality, safety, efficiency and cost of drugs and equipments are important considerations in choosing an anaesthetic technique for outpatient surgery. It should have rapid and smooth onset of action and should produce intraoperative amnesia, analgesia, good surgical conditions and with short recovery period without any side effects.

The choice of anaesthetic technique depends on both surgical and patient's factor. For many ambulatory surgeries general anaesthesia remains the most popular technique. Central neuronal blockade has been useful for peripheral procedures but it delays the discharge of patient due to prolonged sympathetic blockade.

Now a days, the procedures are performed with a combination of local nerve blocks and intravenous sedation, called as monitored anaesthesia care technique.

Monitored Anaesthesia Care

The combination of local anaesthetic with intravenous analgesic and sedative drugs is gaining popularity in ambulatory surgery. This technique was introduced by American Dental Association and called as Conscious sedation. This has rapid recovery with less side effects.

Office–based Anaesthesia

It is a variant of ambulatory anaesthesia which has attracted growing interest for short surgical procedures. As efforts to reduce the overall cost of surgical procedures continue to increase, Surgeon and Anaesthesiologists are transferring the cases to facilities where these have more direct control over cost.

Anaesthesia for procedures outside operating room

Anaesthesiologists are being called upon to provide anaesthetic care for an increasing number of procedures in remote locations. The most common are Electro – convulsive therapy (ECT), Extra – corporal shock wave lithotripsy (ESWL), neurodiagnostic procedures such as Magnetic resonance imaging (MRI) and computed tomography (CT).

Here in all these procedures one has to confirm the technical problems, surgical technique intra and postoperative related complications.

The anaesthesia machine and monitors are not in frequent use, expert assistants are not available or nursing staff is not adequate and there is un – accustomed environment. In these situations, the patient must be carefully selected and evaluated prior to the procedure. The anaesthesia technique should provide a prompt recovery with minimal side effects. May of these procedures have specific anaesthetic consideration and potential complications, which may require careful management.

Discharge Criteria

There are three stages of recovery following ambulatory surgery namely, early, intermediate and late.

- Early recovery is the time interval during which patients emergence from anaesthesia, recover their protective reflexes and resume motor activity. During the phase of recovery, vital signs and oxygen saturation are carefully monitored and supplements of oxygen, analgesics and anti-emetics may be given. The Aldvete score is commonly used to assess the fitness to be transferred to phase II recovery.
- During the intermediate recovery period, patients are for in a reclining chair and progressively begin to ambulate, drink fluids, void and prepare for discharge.
- The late recovery starts when the patient is discharged home and continues until full functional recovery is achieved and able to return to work. The surgical procedure itself has the impact on patient's full functional recovery.

The availability of rapid and short acting anaesthetic drugs for the maintainance of anaesthesia (Propofol, Desflurane or Sevofurane) has facilitated the early recovery of outpatients after ambulatory surgical procedures. A faster early recovery may not necessarily correlate the major determinants of postanasethesia care unit (PACU), cost is personnel. However, significant cost saving may be achieved by bypassing the PACU and transferring patients directly to a more economical phase II (step down) recovery area. There is growing interest.

In this process known as fast tracking after ambulatory surgery.

The Post – Anaesthetic discharge Scoring System (PADSS) is simple cumulative index that measures patient's home readiness and is based on five measure criteria :

- Vital signs – including blood pressure, heart rate, respiratory rate and temperature.
- Ambulation and mental state
- Pain and postoperative nausea and vomiting (PONV)
- Surgical bleeding
- Fluid intake and output.

Modified Post-anaesthesia Discharge Scoring System :

Vital Signs

- 2 – Within 20% of preoperative value
- 1 – 20–40 % of preoperative value
- 0 – 40% of preoperative value

Ambulation

- 2 – Steady gait/no dizziness
- 1 – with assistance
- 0 – none/dizziness

Nausea and Vomiting

- 2 – Minimal
- 1 – Moderate
- 0 – Severe

Pain

- 2 – Minimal
- 1 – Moderate
- 0 – Severe

Surgical bleeding

- 2 – Minimal
- 1 – Moderate
- 0 – Severe

Patients achieving score of 9 or more and have an adult escort are considered fit for discharge.

Patients recovering from regional anaesthesia must meet the same discharge criteria as patients recovering from general anaesthesia.

There is considerable controversy as the requirement for all out patients to drink fluid and void urine prior to discharge from an ambulatory surgical faculty. It is important to have an efficient mechanism for admitting outpatients in the hospital.

As out-patients surgery continues to grow and the types of surgical procedures become more complex, ambulatory surgical centers must develop methods to evaluate patient outcome during both early and late recovery periods. The overall risk of major morbidity and mortality is very low following outpatient surgery.

Unexpected hospital admission following outpatient surgery is an easily identified and important outcome measure in ambulatory anaesthesia. The most common causes for unexpected admission are severe pain, bleeding, intractable vomiting, surgical mishaps, extensive surgery, urinary retention or lack of an adult escort.

The likelihood of admission is related more to the type of surgical procedure and type of anaesthesia than specific patient characteristics. The frequency of return hospital admission after discharge from ambulatory units is another outcome measure.

Predisposing factors for complications during and after outpatient anaesthesia are :

Pre – existing disease
- None ASA – I   1/156
- Diabetis mellitus   1/149
- Bronchial asthma   1/139
- Chronic pulmonary disease   1/112

- Hypertension   1/87
- Heart disease   1/74

Type of Anaesthesia
- Local only   1/268
- Regional only   1/247
- Regional with sedation   1/106
- General anaesthesia   1/120

Duration of Anaesthesia
- Less than 1 hour   1/155
- 1 to 2 hours   1/84
- More than 2 hours   1/54
- More than 3 hours   1/35

Guidelines for Discharge

- Stable vital signs for atleast 1 hour.
- No evidence of respiratory depression or airway obstruction.
- Well oriented in time, place and person.
- Able to dress and walk by its own.
- Able to take fluids orally and void urine.
- Minimal nausea and vomiting.
- Tolerable postoperative pain.
- Responsible adult escort.
- Patient has received instructions of postoperative care.

(K. Korttila, 1989)

A wide variety of psychomotor tests have been used to assess the recovery following general anaesthesia or sedation. Most of these tests are too complex and time consuming to use in busy clinical settings but are of practical importance. The Blender Gestalt Tracker Tracer Test is a reliable, valid, objective, non-invasive, less expensive test that can be easily performed on outpatient within a minute.

Psychomotor Tests

1. **Simple Reaction time :** The time taken to press a button in

response to single light source flashed randomly at a constant place.

2. **Choice reaction time :** The time taken to press the correct button corresponding to one of four colored light sources flashed randomly at four constant places.

3. **Perceptive accuracy test :** The percentage of correct responses in identifying two numbers displayed on a computer screen for 0.5 secs.

4. **Digit substitution test :** The number and percentage of correct substitution of symbols for numbers according to a key within 90 secs.

5. **Bender Gestalt Track Tracer Test :** The percentage of time a stylus is in contact with the side while tracing narrow circular and square track.

6. **Trigger Dot test :** The accuracy of joining dots on paper as judged by the number of dots missed.

(Gupta A etal, 1992)

A major limiting factor in outpatient surgery at present is inadequate postoperative pain management. It is true that, the necessity of day care surgery in our country is more than any developed country but these differ in many aspects.

Developed countries have their own day care societies of Anaesthesiologists to hold regular meetings with aim and discussion of problems related to day care surgery. These have even regular educational meetings amongst hospital personnel, community health centers and general practioners.

Summary

Ambulatory anaesthesia is continuing to evolve and has now become a recognized anaesthesia specialty with formal postgraduate teaching programme.

It is clear than the number of operations performed on an outpatient basis will continue to expand in the 21st century.

Increasing evidence suggests that arbitury limits placed on the type of surgery, age of patient, duration of the operation and preoperative fasting period may be unwarranted. The ability to provide adequate pain management following outpatient surgery has become a major limiting factor in determining the types of operative procedures that can be performed in this settings.

The expansion of home health care services creates potential problems for newer analgesic modalities to be used at home. With growing limitations on health care resources, the anaesthesiologists must carefully re – evaluate clinical practice. The incidence of anaesthesia related side effects may be altered depending on the premedication, anaesthesia technique and skill of administrator.

Drawbacks

Every one of us since joining the anaesthesia fraternity are practicing day care surgery or ambulatory surgery. This is being carried without knowing much details but it was under minor operative procedures.

One must keep in mind that there might be minor surgical procedure but there is no minor anaesthesia technique. For any type of surgical procedure, either general or regional / local anaesthesia has to be provided. In general anaesthesia, premedication, induction and maintainance and recovery has to be there for any type of surgery. The patient has to preoperatively evaluated for fitness of anaesthesia, intraoperative monitoring and observed for some time postoperatively. The postgraduate students of Anaesthesiology are so trained and advised to practice anaesthesia according to these guidelines. One must not side track the basic concepts for doing anaesthesia practice.

No doubt due to the introduction of new techniques of anaesthesia, new drugs (intravenous inducing agents, inhalational anaesthetic agents, sedatives, analgesics, muscle relaxants and local anaesthetic agents) and more important recent developments in surgical technology, one has to be ready to accept recent concepts of anaesthesia practice.

To accept the new challenges in technology, the academicians or teaching staff members has to educate and train the postgraduates of Anaesthesiology accordingly.

The main problem is that, the Government medical institutes

are not having all the facilities of training the postgraduate students, as well as there is always scarcity of new drugs just introduced in the practice. The equipment facilities, teaching staff members, operation theater updating, postoperative care, etc are not upto the standard to fulfill the demands of ambulatory surgery.

Previous academic devotion, teaching interest of senior staff is also lacking and the interest in learning of the students is not satisfactory. All these are the contributory factors for to have more concern in this new concept of day care surgery.]

This problem can be some how diluted by developing the interest in postgraduates as well as provoking them for attending various workshops, CME, seminars and conferences of Anaesthesiology and also axillary branches of Anaesthesiology. This will help for learning them, updating the knowledge and educated for practice of good day care surgery.

Another aspect of this day care surgery is the non – availability of new equipments, drugs that are essential in recent technology of surgery and accordingly our anaesthesia practice should be updated. Always there is short of funds for purchase of new equipments and drugs in government ruined medical institutes. Our society should take efforts to convince the government for fulfilling our requirements for practicing day care surgery.

The state governments should be made aware of the cost benefits encored on every patient after hospital admission and after day care surgery.

Illiteracy in the patients and the relatives about merits and demerits of day care surgery is also main problem in its success. As more than 60% of our population resides in rural areas and there is ignorance about own health. Even now these people believe on vaidhya and mantras. The peoples should be educated about the importance of preoperative anaesthesia evaluation, these should inform about the addictions, drug therapy, previous medical illness, preoperative fasting and postoperative care in relation to technique of ambulatory surgery.

The transportation facility for the approach to medical aid is not there so the transport inconvience for day care surgery is out of reach. The primary health centers, rural and civil hospitals and medical institutes are not well equipped to fulfill the requirements of day care surgery.

At metro politan cities or big cities, though day care surgery is routinely practiced but here also there are no facilities or follow up of patients in postoperative period. The peoples should be educated about early reporting of the postoperative complications after day care surgery.

The surgeons are many times over enthusiastic about the application of day care surgery but the Anaesthesiologists must confirm the facilities, resources available, postoperative outcome and finally his efficiency in the practice of day care surgery. One must see the applicability of the technique in concern with safety rather than facing the complications itself. One must get acquainted with the new techniques and drugs first before actual practice. It is not safe to use the new techniques only after reading the literature or already use in developed countries but get education of that and then use.

On first sight, the day care surgery looks to have many merits in all aspects as time factor, cost benefit, economical in patient's view, comfort but on the other hand the main draw back is less knowledge about its applicability, monitoring aids and postoperative care.

Again, non-availability of funds for full set up of day care unit, equipments, drugs, surgical technology, transport facility, communication and patients awareness, ignorance of relatives, all contribute to less popularity of day care surgery in India.

Education of the lay man, relatives, patient, nursing staff, paramedical persons and even practicing anaesthesiologists may update future of ambulatory or day care surgery is necessary.

14

Cardio-Pulmonary Resuscitation

One of the commonest health and hospital emergencies is that of cardio-pulmonary arrest with the interruption of Oxygen system. Restoration of the cardiac activity and establishment of tissue oxygen supply should be the immediate goal.

Definition : Cardiac arrest is sudden failure of cardiac action and due to either asystole or ventricular fibrillation.

In general causes of cardiac arrest include :

- Ischemic heart disease
- Drowning
- Electrocution
- Suffocation
- Drug intoxication
- Automobile accidents

1. Basic Life support

It is the emergency first aid procedure that consists of the recognition of airway obstruction, respiratory arrest, cardiac arrest and proper application of cardio-pulmonary resuscitation.

CPR consists of :

- Opening and maintaining patient's airway
- Providing artificial ventilation by means of rescue breathing

- Providing artificial circulation by means of external cardiac compression

2. Advanced life support

It is basic life support with use of adjunctive equipments, intravenous fluid lifeline (infusion) drug administration, defibrillation, stabilization of victim by cardiac monitoring, control of Dysarrhythmias and post-resuscitation care.

Indications of Resuscitation are :

a) Respiratory arrest

b) Cardiac arrest :

- Cardiovascular collapse (electro-mechanical dissociation
- Ventricular fibrillation
- Ventricular standstill or asystole

Basic life support is an emergency first aid procedure. A maximum sense of urgency is required. It includes A–B–C steps of cardio-pulmonary resuscitation.

Heart Lung Resuscitation (HLR)

or

Cardio-pulmonary Resuscitation

Principles	*Personnel*
A Airway	Non-medical
B Breathing	Paramedical
C Circulation	
D Definitive	
D : Diagnosis	Medical
D : Drugs	
D : Defibrillation	
D : Disposition	

These steps should be started as quickly as possible. These are different in monitored patients or in witnessed cardiac arrest. When the cardiac arrest occurs in the monitored patient, trained personnel and defibrillator are available immediately, precordial thump and or advanced life support procedures should be instituted without delay. In a witnessed cardiac arrest, A–B–C sequence should include use of precordial thump.

Respiratory inadequacy may result from an obstruction of the airway or from respiratory failure. An obstructed airway is difficult to recognize until the airway is opened. A partially obstructed airway is recognized by labored breathing or excessive respiratory effort involving accessory muscles of respiration, soft tissue retraction of the intercostals, supraclavicular and suprasternal spaces.

Respiratory failure is characterized by minimal or absent respiratory effort, failure or upper abdominal movements and inability to detect air through nose or mouth.

Opening of airway and restoring breathing are basic steps of artificial ventilation. The steps can be performed quickly under almost any circumstances and without adjunctive equipments or help of another person.

Establishment of Airway

- The initial and most important procedure of successful resuscitation is immediate opening of airway.
- Tilt head backwards as far as possible. This maneuver opens up the pharynx and it is effective in most of cases.
- Chin lift : Pulling chin forward will improve the passage way by further advancing tongue forward away from the pharynx.
- Jaw thrust : additional opening of the airway or passage may be achieved by forward displacement of jaw at the angle of mandible. When trained personnel are present airway or 'S' shaped airway can be inserted.
- Often maneuvers to establish a clear airway result in patient breathing. When establishment of airway does not result in the victim resuming spontaneous breathing, the rescuer must move to provide artificial ventilation.

Artificial Ventilation

a) Mouth to mouth ventilation
b) Mouth to nose ventilation – when it is difficult to open the mouth and impossible to ventilate via mouth due to facial injury then one must try mouth to nose ventilation.
c) Direct mouth to stoma
d) Self inflating bag and mask or machine – After temporarily starting or assisting ventilation, when patient can not continue his breathing efforts then patient is kept on mechanical ventilators.

Precipitating factors in sudden cardiac collapse

I) **Factors initiating neuro-muscular reflexes :**

Efferent vagal stimulation – from thoracic and cervical region

Vasovagal reflexes

Any efferent stimulus with vagal efferent pathway

- Pain – skin
- Anal dilatation
- Pharyngo-tracheal stimulation
- Periosteum – bone fractures
- Visceral traction

II) **Chemical factors and anaesthesia :** Hypoxia, hypercarbia, asphyxia, adrenal secretions, non-anaesthetic drugs, over doses of anaesthetic agents and errors in technique.

III) **Physical and Physiological factors :**

- Anomalies : diaphragmatic hernia, congenital cardiac defects
- Cardiac tamponade
- Torsion, pressure or retraction of heart or adjacent structures
- Abnormal or sudden changes in surgical position
- Preoperative hypovolumia
- Hyperthermia
- Miscellaneous

IV) **Surgical factors :**
- Site of surgery – intra-thoracic, intra-abdominal, intra-cranial
- Major and prolonged surgery
- Blood loss

V) **Factors during anaesthesia :**
- Cardio-vascular
- Severe uncontrolled hypotension
- Air embolism
- Myocardial infarction
- Dysarrhythmias
- Respiratory factors :
- Airway obstruction, secretions, laryngospasm
- Aspiration
- Failure to intubate – difficult intubation, oesophageal intubation, accidental extubation
- Carbon dioxide retention
- Post-extubation airway obstruction
- Pneumothorax
- Physiological criteria of Respiratory failure
- Respiratory rate - more than 35
- Vital capacity – less than 15 ml / kg
- FEV_1 – less than 10 ml / kg
- Inspiratory force – less than 25 cm H_2O
- PaO_2 – less than 70 mm of Hg
- $PaCO_2$ – more than 55 mm of Hg
- VD/VT – more than 0.60

Anatomical and Physiological factors affecting Normal Alveolar Ventilation and causing acute Respiratory failure :

1. **Respiratory Centre :**
   - Circulatory shock

- Increased intra-cranial pressure
- Increase or decrease in PaO_2
- Narcotic analgesics

2. **Motor-neuron connection :**
   - Phrenic nerve disruption
   - Upper motor neuron disease
   - Polio myelitis
   - Poly neuritis – anterior horn cells
   - Lower motor neuron disease

3. **Neuro-muscular junction :**
   - Myasthenia gravis
   - Muscle relaxants
   - Botulism
   - Neostigmine over doses

4. **Respiratory muscles :**
   - Muscular dystrophies
   - Injury to diaphragm
   - Over distended abdomen

5. **Lung and chest wall elasticity :**
   - Emphysema
   - ARDS
   - Pulmonary edema
   - Pneumonitis

6. **Patency of airway :**
   - Upper airway obstruction
   - Status asthmaticus

7. **Bony cage and Pleural cavity :**
   - Pneumothorax
   - Flail chest
   - Lung collapse
   - Alveolar edema

Artificial Circulation

- External cardiac compression
- Precordial thump
- Internal cardiac compression
- Defibrillation or cardio version

When sudden, unexpected cardiac arrest occurs, all of A–B–C of basic life support are required in rapid succession. This includes both artificial circulation and artificial ventilation.

Cardiac arrest is diagnosed by pulselessness in large arteries in an unconscious victim and absent breathing. In an unwitnessed, the rescuer must first open the airway and quickly ventilate the lungs, carotid or femoral pulse is usually palpated.

External Cardiac compression

- For effective external cardiac compression, the victim must be on a firm surface in a horizontal position.
- Feel the tip of xiphoid and place the long axis of heel of one hand parallel to and over long axis of the lower 1/3 to ½ of the sternum. Place the other hand on top of first hand (interlock the fingers)
- Bring the shoulders directly over the victim's chest. Keep the arms straight and exert pressure almost vertically downwards to depress the lower sternum a minimum of 1.5" to 2" towards spine. The compression must be regular, rhythmic, smooth and uninterrupted.
- Relaxation must immediately follow compression of equal duration. The heel of hand should not be removed in between the relaxation period but pressure must be completely released, so the sternum returns to normal position. This permits full re-expansion of the lungs and filling of vascular tissues in the chest.
- The compression rate for 2 rescuers is 60 /minute. This rate produces a systolic blood pressure of 70 mm of Hg.
- When there is one rescuer, then must perform both artificial

ventilation and artificial circulation using 15 : 2 ratio, two quick lung inflations after each 15 chest compressions.

- In small children, heel of one hand or tips of index and middle fingers are used, kept at mid-sternum area. The compression rate should be 80 – 100 per minute with breaths delivered as quickly as possible after each 5 compressions.

Effectiveness of CPR

The reaction of pupils should be checked periodically during CPR, as this provides best indication of Oxygenation. Reaction of pupils indicate adequate oxygenation and blood flow to brain. The carotid pulse should be palpated periodically during CPR so that effectiveness can be assessed.

Precordial Thump

- Precordial thump is used in witnessed cardiac arrest (basic life support) monitored patient (advanced life support), pacing and known atrio-ventricular block (advanced life support).
- Precordial thump is not recommended in Paediatric patients :
- In cases where primary cause of cardiac arrest is not hypoxia, a single precordial thump may be effective in restoring cardiac action and may reverse some Dysarrhythmias.
- It may be effective in restoring beats in ventricular asystole due to block, ventricular tachycardia or fibrillation.
- Precordial thump should be sharp, quick, single blow over mid portion of sternum form 8" to 12" over the chest with ulnar border of palm.
- Deliver the thump within first minute of cardiac arrest. When there is no immediate response, then begin basic life support.

Precautions in Performance of CPR

- Do not interrupt CPR for more than 5 seconds except if endotracheal intubation is already performed.
- Do not move the patient until stabilization and ready for

transportation so that un-interrupted CPR during movement is provided.

- Do not compress the xiphoid process at the tip of sternum as laceration of liver can occur.
- In between compressions, release the pressure of hand.
- Body of rescuer should not press the ribs.
- Compression should be smooth, regular and uninterrupted.
- Do not maintain continuous pressure on abdomen.
- The shoulders of rescuer should be directly over the victim's sternum. The elbows should be straight and pressure is applied vertically downwards on lower sternum.
- Usual CPR may result in complications as fracture of ribs, fracture of sternum, costo-chondral separation, Pneumothorax, haemothorax, lung contusion, laceration of liver and fat embolism.
- Special situations are – Drowning, Electric shock and chocking syndrome.

Internal Cardiac compression

When chest is already open, then heart (ventricles) is grasped in between thumb rested at the base of heart inferiorly and index and middle finger at the opposite side of thumb superiorly, or heart is squeezed in the fist of palm. The ventricles are squeezed as quickly as possible within 1 second. This is performed for about 60 – 80 times per minute. It is effective for circulation.

Advanced Life Support

Advanced Life support consists of :

1. **Initial Basic life support :**
   - Use of adjunctive equipments, special technique as endotracheal intubation and open chest internal cardiac compression.
   - Recognition of Dysarrhythmias and control
   - Defibrillation

- Establishment and maintainance of intravenous infusion lifeline
- Employing definitive therapy as correction of acidosis, maintainance of effective cardiac rhythm and circulation.
- Stabilization of patient's condition.

2. **Internal cardiac compression :** When chest is already open or in situations like tension Pneumothorax, flail chest, multiple fractures of ribs, haemothorax, it is useful. It is performed along with artificial ventilation of lungs.

3. **Cardiac monitoring :** ECG monitoring to detect the type of cardiac arrest as sinus arrest or ventricular fibrillation or various arrhythmias.

4. **Defibrillation :** Defibrillation produces simultaneous depolarization at all muscles fascicles of heart after which a spontaneous beat may resume when myocardium is well oxygenated and not acidotic. Direct current defibrillator shocks should be delivered as soon as possible in ventricular fibrillation.

   The standard electrode position should be used- one electrode is placed just right of upper sternum below clavicle and other is placed just left to apex of heart or left nipple. 150 – 200 joules current is given at one time and can be repeated. In paediatric patients 1–2 joules/kg current is used.

5. **Intravenous therapy :** It is essential to provide an intravenous route for
   - Intermittent or continuous rapid administration of drugs and fluids may be required to re-establish or support stable cardiac rhythm and adequate circulation

6. **Drugs and definitive therapy :**
   - Oxygen and ventilation.
   - Essential drug therapy – Epinephrine, Sodium bicarbonate, Hydrocortisone, etc.

7. **Special Drug therapy :**
   - Atropine sulphate
   - Lignocaine hydrochloride

- Calcium chloride
- Metaraminol (vasoactive drug)
- Isoprenaline
- Propranolol
- Corticosteroids
- Post-cardiac arrest drug therapy – In addition to Corticosteroids, potent diuretics, hypotension and controlled hyperventilation may be useful for prevention and attenuation of cerebral edema, which is usually follow successful resuscitation.

Termination of life support

- It depends upon an assessment by Physician of cerebral status of the patient. The best criteria of adequate cerebral circulation are reaction of pupils, level of consciousness, movement of extremities and spontaneous respiration.
- Deep unconsciousness, absent spontaneous respiration, fixed and dilated pupils for 15–30 minutes are usually indications of cerebral death and there is no need for continuation of further resuscitation.
- Cardiac death is recognized as absence of electro-cardio graphic activity upto 10 minutes after arrest.

Contraindications of Resuscitation

- In cases of terminal ir-reversible illness
- When the time from cardiac arrest is more than 10 – 15 minutes
- When arrest is outside hospital as exact time of arrest can not be available.

Definitive Therapy in Cardiac Resuscitation

	Diagnosis
Definitive	Drugs
	Defibrillation

I. Diagnosis

- Cardiac standstill – Absent heart beat , flat ECG
- Ventricular fibrillation – uncoordinated heart beats, erratic activity on ECG
- Cardiovascular collapse – Rhythmic or ineffective heart beats, ECG may be normal,
- For all these signs are with absent breathing, absent pulse and dilated pupils.

Always continue heart-lung resuscitation without interruption during diagnosis

II. Drugs

1. **Epinephrine :** 0.5–1 ml (1:1000), improves blood pressure and cardiac tone
2. **Sodium bicarbonate :** 1 ml/kg–corrects acidosis and improves cerebral blood flow.
3. **Calcium chloride :** Upto 10 ml (10%)–increases myocardial tone and increases cardiac output.
4. **Vasopressors :** After restoration of heart beats
5. **Qunidine or Procaine amide :** 100 mg – decreases myocardial irritability

Always continue heart-lung resuscitation without interruption during administration of drugs.

III. Defibrillation

- Use external defibrillation – 30 pounds pressure on electrodes over saline pads in standard position.
- AC : 440–880 volts, DC : 100–200 volts/sec.
- Repeat shocks, repeat drugs.

Always continue heart-lung resuscitation without interruption between defibrillation.

15

Postoperative Anaesthetic Complications

The patients undergoing emergency surgery are particularly prone to develop complications in the postoperative period. Inadequate preparation and various untreated associated medical disorders prose problems for smooth intra-operative course of anaesthesia and postoperative recovery. Hence, the incidence postoperative complications is relatively less in elective operative procedures due through preoperative evaluation and preparation of the patients. Again the incidence of postoperative complications is more in emergency obstetric and trauma patients as compared to any other emergency operative procedures. These postoperative complications mainly after emergency surgery are considered under following headings –

1. Inadequate Respiration
2. Delayed recovery of consciousness
3. Postoperative hypotension
4. Various arrhythmias
5. Pulmonary complications

INADEQUATE RESPIRATION

Emergency patients particularly receiving general anaesthesia are prone to develop respiratory inadequacy postoperatively. This may be in the from of prolonged aponea, obvious respiratory impairment and respiratory acidosis.

Inadequate respiration may be due to defects in respiratory mechanism as gaseous exchange fails to maintain the normal level of arterial Oxygen and Carbon dioxide tensions. The fault may be in central nervous system, myoneural junction or due to pre-existing or recent deterioration in pulmonary functions.

The assessment of postoperative respiratory functions is difficult and most of the methods are inappropriate in immediate postoperative period.

Visual evidence of inadequate respiration can be obtained by observing pattern and type of breathing.

Presence of tracheal tug or jerky diaphragmatic respiration with pause after inspiration is indicative of incomplete reversal after muscle relaxants or carbon dioxide retention.

A slow, shallow respiration is usually due to central depression secondary to over doses of sedatives, narcotic analgesics, intravenous or inhalational anaesthetic agents or intra-cranial pathology.

Use of accessory muscles of respiration is indicative of inadequate respiratory functions.

Tidal volume is not good indicator of respiratory functions but minute volume readings taken at various time intervals confirm apparent improvement in ventilation postoperatively.

Estimation of arterial Carbon dioxide is an accurate index of respiratory efficacy. Serial readings of Pco_2 at hourly intervals will provide accurate guide to trend respiratory adequacy.

A rising pulse rate and blood pressure in patients who are sweating, anxious, restless and purposeless movements often denote Carbon dioxide retention and early hypoxia due to inadequate ventilation.

There are many causes of inadequate postoperative respiration particularly in unprepared, dehydrated, seriously ill patients where more than one factor is responsible. The respiratory impairment may be due to :

• Central nervous system

- Peripheral neuromuscular block
- Mechanical factors
- Metabolic acidosis

Central nervous system

One of the cause of inadequate respiration following general anaesthesia is failure of respiratory center, this may be due to depression by drugs, injury or lack of afferent stimuli.

- Central depression is more likely to cause inadequate respiration mainly after emergency procedure than after elective operations. Improper preoperative assessment, busy schedule or improper administration of sedatives and narcotic analgesics as premedication without individual differentiation may cause postoperative central depression. These problems are more serious in patients with hypotension and peripheral circulatory failure.

- Inhalational anaesthetic agents like Cyclopropane, Halothane have marked respiratory depression action. Narcotic analgesics like Morphine, Pethidine, Buperonorphine when used intermittently for intra-operative analgesia may result in central respiratory depression postoperatively. Cumulative effects of drugs, relative over doses with aponea, severe depression or slow respiration are results of mis-management. The problems do occur in patients with Myoxedema, Porphyria, Muscular dystrophy and Dystrophica myotonica.

- Depression of respiratory center may also occur in presence of peripheral circulatory failure, following severe hypoxic episodes. Central depression rarely may occur due to cerebrovascular accidents, extradural or subdural haematoma, head injury, hyperpyrexia, convulsions due to any cause, etc.

Hyperventilation : It lowers the arterial PCo_2 and remove normal stimulus to respiratory center.

Hypoventilation results in Carbon dioxide retention and cause respiratory inadequacy postoperatively. Carbon dioxide retention may occur due to exhausted Soda lime, under ventilation by administrator, distended abdomen, raised diaphragm, pulmonary secretions, bronchospasm, chronic bronchitis, emphysema, congestive cardiac failre, etc all results in hypoventilation.

Habit and Reflex aponea : It is some times present after prolonged periods of controlled ventilation. Habit aponea may be due to exhaustion of Hering Bruer reflex.

Peripheral Neuro-muscular Block

Prolonged aponea due to non-depolarizing muscle relaxants, inadequate reversal and respiratory inadequacy may occur postoperatively. This may be due to relative over dose, true sensitivity, electrolyte imbalance, antibiotics, mismanagement and mixed block.

Prolonged aponea may occur in debilated patients, poor cardiac out put states, haemorrhagic shock, prolonged hypotension, dehydration, stagnant peripheral circulation, electrolyte imbalance, hypokalemia, upper gastro-intestinal obstruction, vomiting, paralytic ileus, renal disease, mycin group of antibiotics, will all result in inadequate reversal of neuro-muscular block and postoperative respiratory inadequacy in emergency patients.

Mismanagement during intra-operative period – improper drug administration, mixed block, prolonged aponea after Suxamethonium secondary to low levels of pseudocholinesterase, dual block, excess production of Succinyl monocholine, all will result in respiratory inadequacy in postoperative period.

Mechanical Impairment

Disturbances of pulmonary functions can occur due to respiratory obstruction such as laryngeal oedema, pulmonary aspiration, bronchospasm, pulmonary oedema, Pneumothorax, fracture ribs or presence of restrictive/obstructive airway diseases may result in postoperative respiratory inadequacy.

4. Metabolic acidosis

Metabolic acidosis occur when non-volatile acids accumulate in the body as a result of Diabetic coma, hypoxia, trauma, severe hypotension or diarrhoea. The condition is aggravated when normal compensatory mechanisms of renal adjustment, hyperventilation, failure of elimination of carbon dioxide will not correct the acidosis.

Hypokalaemia, over doses of muscle relaxants, carbon dioxide retention. Mixed block, all will enhance metabolic acidosis and result in respiratory inadequacy.

Prolonged intestinal obstruction, clamping of large blood vessels for longer time, cardiac arrest, peripheral circulatory failure and hypotension are main causes of metabolic acidosis and respiratory inadequacy. The correction of metabolic acidosis automatically improves the respiration of patient postoperatively.

Management of inadequate respiration

- Adequate and complete reversal on neuro-muscular block
- Assisted ventilation even after extubation
- Avoid reflex stimulation of upper airway
- Frequent estimation of PCO_2
- Frequent estimation of serum electrolytes
- Correction of metabolic acidosis

Correct central depression – by watching the respiration and appropriate antidote administration when required, only assist the respiration till the effect of drugs is weaned off.

Establishment of clear airway or correction of bronchospasm and ventilation should clear mechanical impairment according to cause.

For correction of respiratory inadequacy the exact causative factor should be checked, assessed and corrected accordingly. It requires patience and immediate intervention so that patient will not develop permanent damage.

DELAYED RECOVERY OF CONSCIOUSNESS

The use of modern anaesthesia techniques and newer drugs have reduced the chances of delayed recovery of consciousness postoperatively, even in emergency patients. Now a days it is only observed in critically ill patients, untreated patients for associated medical disorders, surgical or anaesthesia accidents or idiosyncrasy.

The possible causes of postoperative delayed recovery or coma are :

- Cerebral hypoxia
- Carbon dioxide retention
- Metabolic acidosis
- Anaesthesia over doses
- Associated severe medical disorders
- Irreversible Shock
- Cerebo-vascular accidents
- Fat embolism or amniotic fluid embolism
- Hypothermia

Cerebral hypoxia

The post-operative patients with coma have stertorous or gasping respiration, dilated pupils and motor in-coordinate movements of extremities following hypoxic episode or cardiac arrest is obviously suffering from residual cerebral damage and urgent dehydration treatment is indicated. The therapy will reduce cerebral oedema resulting from hypoxic capillary damage. The oedema fluid acts as a physical barrier to Oxygen diffusion, intra-cranial tension is raised, respiration is depressed, it increases in intensity to cause irreversible damage and cell death.

As a result hypoxia may develop secondary to anoxia, anaemia, Stagnant or histotoxic hypoxia or in combination. Hypoxia is less likely to be imputed as a causative factor and failure to initiate early treatment may prejustice patients for complete recovery.

Delayed recovery of consciousness is more suggestive , a relapse into coma after some hours of semi-consciousness or confusion is enough to raise the possibility of hypoxic damage. Intra-operative laryngeal spasm, aspiration of vomitus, under ventilation, bronchospasm or respiratory obstruction will cause cerebral hypoxia or in case of severe hypotension due to trauma, shock or haemorrhage. It is usually treated by 50 ml of 50% Dextrose, 100 ml of 25% Mannitol and 4 – 8 mg of Dexamethasone (Efcorlin). In severe cerebral hypoxia may have some Carbon dioxide retention, metabolic acidosis and are treated accordingly.

Carbon dioxide retention

Hypercapnia alone can cause postoperative coma without any hypoxic element. Inadequate preoperative treatment of chest infection as in chronic bronchitis, emphysema, abdominal distension, shock, debility, all predispose inadequate respiratory exchange. Cerebral depressant drugs, bronchospasm, inadequate controlled ventilation, defective CO_2 absorption and incomplete reversal of muscle relaxants will lead to reduced alveolar ventilation and Carbon dioxide retention.

Narcosis develop at PCO_2 level is 80–90 mm of Hg and pH falls below 7.25. Clinically CO_2 retention can be detected by flushing, rapid pulse, elevated blood pressure, pause after inspiration as well as after expiration, jerky movements, tracheal tug, etc. The patient should be hyper-ventilated with a high flow of gases through fresh soda lime. The treatment of cause will automatically treat the CO_2 retention and improve the consciousness.

Metabolic acidosis

Prolonged postoperative coma due to biochemical disturbances occurs. It is most commonly encountered after operations as intestinal obstruction and coma from respiratory acidosis, marked hypotension, central respiratory depression, pallor and peripheral cyanosis will be present. There is low pH with low bicarbonate in metabolic acidosis.

Anaesthetic over doses

Delayed recovery of consciousness will occur with normal doses of intravenous inducing agents, inhalational anaesthetic agents and muscle relaxants in critically ill patients, dehydration, cachexia, etc. The over doses should be avoided in these patients.

Anaesthesia and Medical Diseases and Drugs

Severe Liver and Kidney diseases may interfere with de-toxification and excretion of normal doses of anaesthetic agents. Delayed recovery of consciousness is encountered in patients with myoxedema, diabetes, Porphyria, muscular dystrophies, Addisons' disease, daily administration of tranquillizers like Phenothiazines group (Chlorpromazine, Promazine) may prolong the effect of anaesthetic agents, Monoamino oxidase inhibitors (iproiazid, Phenelzine, Tramylcyproine, Isocarboxazid, Nilamide) have potentiating effect on Pethidine and Morphine, when used as premedication. Prolonged coma, severe hypotension, tachycardia, convulsions and Cheyne-Stoke respiration may result and some times mortality. MAO inhibitors also provoke abnormal reactions with presser amines and so these should be avoided.

Shock

Delay in the recovery of consciousness after anaesthesia may be due to severe hypotension or peripheral circulatory failure. In emergency cases it may be due to hypovolumia from loss of blood or plasma or dehydration with added loss of Potassium and Sodium ions.

The normal response to hypotension is peripheral vasocons-triction when treatment is delayed then vasoconstriction becomes more intense, tissue hypoxia develop and compensatory mechanisms are affected. There is loss of muscle tone results in peripheral vasoconstriction and opening of capillary bed, decrease in venous return, inadequate coronary perfusion and myocardial depression due to fall in cardiac output. Increased capillary permeability permits loss of fluid from circulation and result in hypo-volumic shock, increased viscosity and stasis of blood. The end result is coma, renal failure and irreversible shock.

Cardiovascular disorders

Intra-cerebral haemorrhage is extremely rare postoperative complication but cerebral thrombosis is one of the cause of prolonged postoperative unconsciousness. It is common in elderly patients with atherosclerosis and induced by ganglion blockade and shock. It may occur in patients with atrial fibrillation, concomitant head injury, subdural or epidural haematoma. The clinical features are bradycardia, Cheyne-stokes respiration and unequal pupils. Air embolism is rare cause of unconsciousness postoperatively.

Fat embolism or Amniotic fluid embolism

Fat embolism may follow after fractures of long bones. Cerebral symptoms appear within 48 hours of fracture and consists of unexplained restlessness, irritability, delirium, coma or unconsciousness after anaesthesia. Tachyponea or dysponea, snow-storm appearance on X-ray. Low PO_2, defective gas transfer across alveolocapillary membrane due to alveolar oedema, shunting of blood, etc. Recently fat embolism may be due traumatic stress induced release of cathecholamines which result in free fatty acid mobilization and intra-vascular. The treatment is given to improve capillary flow, large doses of Hydrocortisone to treat inflammatory oedema.

Hypothermia

A fall in body temperature may occur after operation in infants and elderly or myxoedematous patients, visceral exposure during laprotomy and after massive cold blood transfusion. Central depression may directly occur during lower body temperature, also there is slow breakdown of intravenously administered drugs due to circulatory depression. There is associated bradycardia, arrhythmia, hypotension and slow respiratory rate in postoperative period in hypothermic patients. There is regaining of consciousness as the body temperature increases.

POSTOPERATIVE HYPOTENSION

A systolic blood pressure below 90 mm of Hg is one of the commonest postoperative complication in emergency operative procedures. Circulatory efficacy is more deteriorated in patients with previous or co-existing medical disorders.

The maintainance of blood pressure depends on adequate cardiac output, efficient vasomotor tone which may lead to fall in arterial pressure. Postoperative hypotension may be due to cardiovascular, respiratory, pharmacological, neurogenic, hematological or humoral factors with postural or bacteriemic hypotension.

Haematological

The commonest cause of postoperative hypotension is inadequate fluid replacement and depends upon the type of fluid loss. Clinically hypotension from hypovolumia will manifest as – peripheral vasoconstriction, skin becomes pale, cold and moist, veins are collapsed. It results in air hunger, anxiety and restlessness. There may be hypotension without blood or fluid loss as in fat embolism, amniotic fluid embolism, air embolism or pulmonary thrombo-embolism.

Respiratory diseases

The second most common cause of postoperative hypotension is hypoxia. It results in myocardial impairment and capillary damage. Mild chronic hypoxia may have disastrous effect on blood pressure. Airway obstruction from atonic or relaxed tongue, upper airway secretions, residual central respiratory depression, inadequate reversal of muscle relaxants or diffusion hypoxia all these conditions which should be prevented. Bronchospasm, aspiration of blood or vomitus, atelectasis, haemo or Pneumothorax and mediastinal shift interferes with respiratory functions. Paradoxical respiration from flail chest rapidly brings about hypoxia, mediastinal flap and hypotension.

Carbon dioxide retention leads to increase in blood pressure due to increased cardiac output and vaso-constriction, this may occur secondary to under ventilation with Cyclopropane and Halothane anaesthesia. Postoperatively as time passes, Anaesthetic concentration decreases, minute volume improves, Co_2 is eliminated, sympathetic stimulation decreases and there may be profound hypotension.

Cardiovascular diseases

Postoperative hypotension may be of cardiac origin. This may be noted in patients with pre-existing valvular disease, cor-pulmonale, hypertension, ischemic heart disease may be decompensated following stress and strain of operation. Arrhythmia as tachycardia develop as a result of toxaemia, hypoxia, electrolyte disturbances or errors of transfusion. Myocardial ischemia or infarction may occur secondary to inadequate coronary perfusion. Some times hypotension may occur in chest injuries due to haemo-pericardium, cardiac tamponade and cardiogenic circulatory failure.

Pharmacological factors

Hypotension may be result of the residual effect of drugs administered in the peri-operative period. It may be due to administration of hypotensive drugs for treatment or control of hypertension, Monoamino oxidase inhibitors (MAO) and Pethidine incompatibility. Bradycardia following Halothane or Neostigmine may result in hypotension. Ganglion blocking drugs, spinal or epidural anaesthesia related sympathetic blockade may cause persistent hypotension in postoperative period also. Injudicious use of Pethidine, Morphine, Phenothiazine derivatives may be responsible for fall in blood pressure in postoperative period.

Neurogenic factors

Certain surgical stimuli in absence of inadequate anaesthesia or light plane of anaesthesia may cause hypotension which persists in the postoperative period. Traction on abdominal viscera, rough handling of intestines may result in hypotension. Fractures of long bones (handling or during reduction) histamine release, toxins from traumatized tissues, peritonitis, ruptured viscera may give rise to persistent hypotension upto postoperative period also.

Vagal tone may be stimulated in recovery period – hypotension and bradycardia results during suction of endotracheal secretions, vomiting, tight dressings, untreated postoperative pain result in restlessness and fall in blood pressure.

Humoral factors

Addison's disease, myoxedema or insulin coma may acuse postoperative hypotension. Adrenocortical atrophy occurs in patients chronically treated with corticostroids and there is deficient response to stress and strain of anaesthesia and surgery and so profound cardiovascular collapse occur.

Postural factors

Residual anaesthesia or postoperative sedation depress the autonomic functions, vasoconstrictive potential is deficient at a time when the harmful effects of many factors upon circulation require full compensatory activity. Rough handling of patient, rolling from side to side to remove strecher or shifting of patient will result in hypotension. A sudden drop in blood pressure may occur when blood is diverted into relatively empty lower limb veins after prolonged periods of lithotomy or Trendelunburg position which should be carried out slowly. Proper care should be taken during these situations and if hypotension results should be treated to avoid cerebral damage due to hypoxia.

Endotoxic shock

Endotoxic shock as a result of gram negative septicemia will cause severe hypotension postoperatively after major intestinal, biliary, urinary tract operations or in severely burn patients. These should be treated with adequate fluid replacement and higher (broad spectrum) antibiotics.

Summary – Treatment of Postoperative Hypotension

- Raising foot end of patient
- Achieving clear airway
- Administration of fluids to correct hypovolumia.
- Drugs :
    - Vasopressors - initially Mephenteramine, nor-adrenaline, Isoprenaline, Ephedrine, etc.
    - α- blocking drugs – Phenoxybenzamine

- Steroids – Hydrocortisone hemisuccinate
- Analgesics – Morphine, Pethidine
- Atropine sulphate
- Calcium gluconate
- Digitalis
- Sodium bicarbonate and 50% Dextrose

CARDIAC ARRHYTHMIAS

The incidence of postoperative arrhythmia is extremely difficult to estimate – many of these are of transient nature, so continuous ECG monitoring is required to detect pathological arrhythmias. True arrhythmias after elective can occur in 1% of cases, after thoracic surgery 12% of patients, following anaesthesia and emergency surgery 5% each, in elderly, pre-existing cardiac disease and circulatory effects of electrolyte and volume disturbances may persist upto postoperative period.

Tachycardia

Sinus reactive tachycardia exists when pulse rate is from 100–150 beats/minute. It is usually compensatory measure and it is important to detect the cause for proper treatment. In the postoperative period, common causes of tachycardia are :

- Residual effects of drugs as Gallamine, Ganglion blocking agents, Atropine, Methyl amphetamine, etc.
- Hypoxia or Hypercarbia due to respiratory obstruction, under ventilation, Pneumothorax, atelectasis, chest injury
- Hypovolumia due to haemorrhage or dehydration, anemia
- Electrolyte imbalance hypokalaemia, metabolic acidosis
- Fever due to toxaemia or septicemia
- Postoperative inadequate pain relief
- Adrenal insufficiency
- Early congestive cardiac failure
- Myocarditis, cardiac tamponade, haemo-pericardium

- Thyroid crisis
- Treatment is the treatment of cause. Some times Digitalization may be necessary or one can try Neostigmine or Procainamide.

Sinus Bradycardia

A pulse rate as low as 60 beats/minute is some times physiological but less than that is pathological. It is manifestation of varying vagal tone and noted with phases of respiration – a slight quickening during inspiration and slowing during expiration. The causes are :

- Occur normally in young adults – vagotonic subjects
- Residual effects of Halothane, Cyclopropane, Neostigmine, Methoxamine, Digitalis, etc.
- Arterio-scelorotic patients have sensitive carotid sinus reflex as in postoperative cervical haematoma, tight dressing or A-V block
- Increased vagal tone noted during recovery of consciousness
- Increase in intra-cranial pressure due to any cause
- Hypotension precipitating posterior myocardial infarction
- Jaundice, Myxoedema, hypothermia
- Bradycardia may itself be corrected, some times Atropine, Isoprenaline, Adrenaline and rarely pace maker may be required for treatment.

Premature beats or Extra systoles

These produce an irregular pulse of variable rate. These may be of atrial or ventricular origin giving rise to pulsus bigeminus. These are diagnosed clinically and confirmed on ECG. Premature beats can occur normally in some individuals, common in elderly patients, residual effects of Halothane or Cyclopropane anaesthesia, Hypercapnia, after Digitalis therapy, myocardial infarction and early congestive cardiac failure. When the ectopic beats are very frequent, treated with Procainamide, Lignocaine. Ventricular extra systoles may occur as result of sudden lowering of raised Pco_2 and there is danger of ventricular tachycardia.

Atrial Fibrillation

Atrial fibrillation produces an irregular tachycardia of 120–150 beats/minute with a variable volume. It almost denotes organic heart disease of ischemic, hypertensive or valvular type. This arrhythmia is common after thoracic surgery in old people may result from hypoxia, hypercarbia, hypotension or mediastinal shift by pleural effusion or atelectasis. It is usually treated with Digitalis. Persistent atrial fibrillation may cause heart failure and interfere with diastolic feeling. Postoperative atrial fibrillation often treated with Digitalis and reverts without DC shock.

Other Arrhythmias

- Atrial flutter, ventricular tachycardia and atrio-ventricular block are rare to occur. These are common in rheumatic, coronary or hypertensive diseases and precipitated with hypoxia, hypercarbia, hypotension and Potassium imbalance.
- Prevention and management of postoperative arrhythmias, anaesthesiologist play an important role.
- Careful management and prompt anaesthetic management.
- Vagal and sympathetic disturbances should be noted early.
- ECG monitoring is necessary for exact diagnosis
- Digitalis therapy in myocardial failure, atrial fibrillation, atrial flutter, atrial tachycardia, elderly patients and congestive cardiac failure.
- Procainamide. Lignocaine, Isoprenaline may be necessary for treatment and lastly DC shock.

PULMONARY COMPLICATIONS

The patients undergoing emergency operations are more prone to develop postoperative chest or pulmonary complications. The common complications are :
- Atelectasis
- Pneumonitis or Bronchopneumonia
- Aspiration Pneumonitis

- Pneumothorax
- Pulmonary fat embolism

Atelectasis

It is the commonest postoperative pulmonary complication may be segmental or basal in distribution but occasionally a lobe or whole lung may become airless and collapsed. The causes are :

- **Airway obstruction :** Obstruction of a bronchus or bronchiole by spasm, mucus, sputum or inhales gastric contents result in alveolar gas absorption and collapse of lung tissue.
- **Postoperative hypoventilation :** During the early post-operative period there is a degree of hypoventilation as a result of residual effect of anaesthesia drugs, immobility, painful abdomen, abdominal distension, thoracic wall injury' Shallow respiration may shift the tidal air up and down a constant pathway and finally may cause atelectasis.
- **Ineffective cough :** Failure to expel secretions add to liability of developing atelectasis. It is common after abdominal emergency surgery, thoracic injury, weakness and exhaustion. Interfere with ability to produce adequate expulsive force to minimize chances of atelectasis.
- **Increased viscosity of secretions :** Ineffective coughing and depression of ciliary activity during early postoperative period impair removal of secretions. It is common after use of Morphine, Pethidine, Atropine, Phenothiazines derivatives which render the sputum more tenacious and difficult to suction.
- Massive collapse of lung is uncommon and occurs on 3rd or 4th postoperative day. The patient often complains of chest pain, dyspnoea, cyanosis, fever, tachycardia, tachypnoea, mediastinal shift, impaired movement of affected lobe, dull percussion note, absent air entry will be clinically noted. The treatment is according to clinical features and symptomatic.

Pneumonitis

It is secondary to infection of atelectic areas. Pyrexia, increased respiratory rate and pallor are noted and with productive cough. Treatment is symptomatic as :

- Inhalation of bronchodilator – Isoprenaline aerosole
- Postural drainage – according to lobe involvement
- Reduction in sputum viscosity by mucolytic agents
- Broad spectrum antibiotics according to culture and sensitivity
- Bronchoscopic aspiration of secretions
- Artificial or mechanical ventilation as when required to avoid hypoxia

Aspiration Pneumonitis

It is common after in patients with full stomach or in all emergency operative procedures particularly in obstetric emergency conditions (caesarean section), trauma, paralytic ileus, intestinal obstruction, road traffic accidents, etc. Prophylaxis is more important than that of treatment.

Pneumothorax

The occurrence of Pneumothorax following emergency anaesthesia may be due to – intercostal drain, chest injury following fracture ribs, para-vertebral block, brachial plexus block, sub-diaphragmatic or cervical surgery, tracheostomy, rupture of emphysematous bulla from inflation pressure during controlled ventilation, CVP cannulation, etc. Tension Pneumothorax may occur when leak is valvular, severe pulmonary and circulatory disturbances follow and urgent treatment is necessary. It is treated with intercostals drainage and Oxygen supplementation.

Pulmonary Fat embolism

It commonly occur after severe bony injury (fractures of long bones). Dyspnoea, tachypnoea, cyanosis, frothy sputum, reduction in arterial Oxygen saturation and the patient detoriates if exact diagnosis and prompt treatment is not under taken immediately. Similar symptoms also noted in amniotic fluid embolism and also in air embolism. It is medical emergency and treated according to the severity of clinical presentation.

MISCELLANEOUS COMPLICATIONS

Shivering

Postoperative shivering is common equally in emergency and elective operative procedures particularly following General anaesthesia with Halothane. Halothane produces peripheral vasodilatation, cold extremities and when patient is suddenly taken out off Halothane administration, there is imbalance between external atmospheric temperature, external lowered body temperature due to vasodilatation and internal body temperature and to cope up with situation, there is increased muscular activity in terms of shivering. It is compensatory mechanism due to increased body metabolism. It is symptomatically treated with Oxygen supplementation and Dextrose infusion.

It may be due to histamine release, anaphylactic or Anaphylactoid reactions, mismatched blood transfusion, hypersensitivity reaction to intravenous fluid as colloids or in cold climate. It is particularly noted in extremes of age as neonates and elderly patients.

Halothane shakes

It is again due to abrupt stoppage of Halothane administration at the end of operative procedure and patient regaining recovery early. Halothane gives rise to peripheral vasodilatation and fall in systemic blood pressure to compensate this, there is increased muscle twitching in the postoperative period. These are a type of involuntary muscle movements called as Halothane shakes which should not be ignored and treated accordingly.

Involuntary movements

Now a days these are very rare due adequate administration of premedicants as sedatives and narcotic analgesics. Some times these may be noted due inadequate pain relief and electrolyte imbalance. Restlessness may be some times presented as involuntary movements.

Nausea and vomiting

It is usually noted following inhalation technique of anaesthesia and during unprepared emergency patients. Postoperative nausea and vomiting is observed in :

- Ether anaesthesia – not commonly used now a days
- Intestinal obstruction
- Obstetric emergency operative procedures
- Acute trauma
- Inadequate reversal or airophasia
- Sub diaphragmatic irritation due to any cause
- During Crash induction and intubation
- One should avoid postoperative nausea and vomiting due likely danger of dreadful complication of aspiration Pneumonitis.

POSTOPERATIVE COMPLICATIONS RELATED TO REGIONAL ANAESTHESIA

Complications of subarachnoid or spinal block

1. Intra-operative

- Failure or dry tap or even drug is injected sometimes there may not be blockade
- High level, hypotension, bradycardia
- Myocardial depression
- Difficulty in respiration due to high level
- Nausea and vomiting
- Tachycardia and hypertension when the block is not adequate
- Sedation due high dose effect of Lignocaine
- Full sensory loss but there may be inadequate muscle relaxation
- Patient complains of uneasiness. So many times the sedative and small doses of narcotics are to be given to get the cooperation of patient

Postoperative complications

- Nausea and vomiting
- Post spinal headache it may either high pressure headache due to meningitis or miningisum and low pressure headache due to leak of CSF there by reducing the CSF pressure causing tension on mininges
- Post operative urinary retention
- Cranial nerve palsy particular VI nerve is common
- Meningitis and miningism
- Transverse myelitis
- Cauda equina syndrome due to adhesive arachnoiditis
- Labyrinthine disturbances
- Backache due use of large size of LP needle
- Anterior spinal artery syndrome
- Total spinal anaesthesia marked hypotension, apnea, dilated pupils, loss of consciousness etc
- Exacerbation of pre-existing spinal cord disease
- Peripheral neuropathy
- Exacerbation of paraesthesia in skin diseases
- Awareness during anaesthesia may have permanent memory on patient and fear of anesthesia in future
- Permanent neurological sequalae
- Pathological fractures in old patients during positioning of patient given for technique
- Injury to spinal cord in paediatric patients as exact anatomical extent of cord can not be localized
- Enthusiastic administration of more fluids in patients to correct hypotension which may cause pulmonary oedema in some patient with fixed output states

Complications of epidural block

- Total subarachnoid block
- Severe hypotension when the block is high

- Severe hypertension if block is inadequate and it is due to pain
- Convulsions or minor muscle twitching
- More chances of failure due to imperfectness
- Inadvertent dural puncture
- Neurological sequalae
- Drowsiness or central depression or sedation
- Hypoapnoea or reduced respiratory rate
- Some times nausea and vomiting
- Patchy effect or patchy analgesia
- Unilateral block due to problem during the position of patient after the administration of drug
- Horner's syndrome
- Headache, vertigo, paraesthesia
- Urinary retention
- Backache due to injury to vertebral column ligaments
- Backache or neck pain due to unaccustomed positioning during administration of block

These complications of spinal or epidural anaesthesia may be in the immediate postoperative period or in the late postoperative period in wards. So to avoid these dreadful complications monitoring of patient in the postoperative period is important and one must not leave the patient as it is done under spinal or epidural or regional anaesthesia. These complications may be noticed in the immediate postoperative period in the recovery room or late in the wards.

The important intraoperative or immediate postoperative complications related to regional anaesthesia is hypersensitivity reaction as rash, urticaria, itching, moderate to severe hypotension, bradycardia and rarely sudden circulatory collapse. This is claimed to be due to preservative present in local anaesthetic solutions. There is histamine release and hypersensitivity reaction. So it is always tested for hypersensitivity reaction before used in any type of regional blocks. It is common with Lignocaine hydrochloride (2%,4% and jelly). With plane Lignocaine (preservative free – there are chances of drug toxicity).

Miscellaneous complications of individual regional blocks

1. Brachial plexus block

- Intra-arterial or intra-venous administration of local anaesthetic agent
- Pneumothorax
- Pleural shock – bradycardia and hypotension – vasovagal stimulation
- Permanent injury to nerves
- Over doses of local anaesthetic agents and toxicity
- Injury to cervical plexus – Horner's syndrome
- Injury to Phrenic nerve – diaphragmatic paralysis
- Injury to recurrent laryngeal nerve - left side
- Failure of block

2. Inter-costal nerve block

- Injury to arterio-venous plexus
- Pneumothorax
- Direct trauma to inter-costal nerve
- Local anaesthetic over doses and toxicity
- Failure of block

3. Cervical plexus block

- Injury to carotid artery, subclavian artery
- Injury to carotid body and sinus
- Injury to internal jugular vein
- Injury to Phrenic, vagus and recurrent laryngeal nerve
- Pneumothorax on right side
- Local anaesthetic over doses and toxicity
- Failure of block

4. Inguinal or Femoral block or Hernia block

- It has less complications
- There are chances of over doses of local anaesthetic agents
- Failure of block

5. Intravenous Regional anaesthesia or Bier's block

- Drug toxicity
- Inadequate analgesia
- Tourniquet pain
- Intra-arterial injection
- Direct injection of local anaesthetic in the arteries through a-v fistula.

16

Role of Anaesthesiologist Outside Operation Theater

INTRODUCTION

The concept of previous working pattern of Anaesthesiologist as to administer required anaesthesia for operative procedures in the operation theater is now totally changed. The working field of anaesthesiologist is widened to a large extent and they are performing the duties to serve human beings in various fields. It is now necessary to get knowledge about the various fields where the anaesthesiologists play a key role. While performing the duties in these fields they have proved their importance in these fields and the vision of other doctors as well as of common man and the patients is totally changed. Again amongst the doctors and particularly at the time of postgraduate choosing options, the trainee doctors are preferring for Anaesthesiology subject as their carrier to serve the patients.

Now a days the anaesthesiologists are concerned in the following fields that are outside the operation theater :

- OPD anaesthesia clinic
- Intensive Respiratory Care Unit
- Intensive Cardiac Care Unit
- Intensive Paediatric Care Unit
- Intensive Neonatal Care Unit

- Intensive Care Unit
- Pain Clinic
- Obstetric analgesia
- Brain Resuscitations
- Cardio-Pulmonary Resuscitation
- Disaster Management
- Psychoanalysis

OPD ANAESTHESIA CLINIC

Screening of the patients for anaesthesia and surgery to be posted for various operative procedures is mandatory in the practice of anaesthesia. Routinely these patients posted for operative procedures are evaluated preanaesthetically for fitness of anaesthesia and surgery in the wards, a day or two prior to surgery. The objectives of preanaesthesia check up are :

- To have conversation with the patient and to allay the anxiety and fear about anaesthesia and surgery amongst the patient and their relatives.
- To detect association of any medical disorder along with surgical pathology in the patients.
- When any medical disorder is present, the status of medical disorder, treatment schedule, drug therapy and any ill effects of the disorder and therapy on other systems.
- To assess for the possibility of impact of medical disorder and drug therapy on technique of anaesthesia, drugs used perioperatively and surgical procedure, etc.
- Advice about routine and specific investigations pertaining to the medical disorder and its significance to conduction of anaesthesia and also to advice about very special and sophisticated investigations if necessary.
- As and when required asking for the Physicians or Specialists opinion for confirmation of diagnosis, treatment and status of physical condition of the patient.
- Particularly in paediatric patients or neonates, one should detect

the association of congenital anomalies or dysfunctions of various systems, etc.

- In female patients one should enquire about obstetric history an history of conception at the time when patient is posted for other surgical pathology than obstetrics.
- In emergency obstetric patients one should evaluate the patients in detail taking into account of physiological changes of pregnancy, association of systemic diseases along with pregnancy, maternal and foetal indications of operative procedures.

All these aspects are mandatory during preanaesthesia evaluation of every patient posted for either elective or emergency operative procedures of any surgical fraternity for smooth conduction of anaesthesia, perioperative period, smooth recovery and less possibility of perioperative morbidity and mortality.

Preoperative assessment for anaesthesia an surgical procedure is usually aimed for :

- Through clinical examination of the patient relevant to anaesthesia and surgery.
- To optimize the physical condition of the patient near to normal, when the patient is having any infective focus in the body should be treated with appropriate antibiotics and anti-histaminic so that patient is fit for anaesthesia and surgery, ex. Upper respiratory tract infection, urinary tract infection, viral fever, etc. Acute attack of bronchial asthma should be treated with broncho-dilators, settled and then accepted.
- Advice about appropriate drug therapy to control or normalize the medical disorders. Anti-hypertensives for control of blood pressure. Anti-arrhythmic for control of arrhythmias, anti-anginal for myocardial ischemia, anti-diabetics for control of blood sugar, anti-thyroid fro hyperthyroidism, anti-tubercuous, blood transfusion for correction of anaemia, etc. Here some drugs should be continued on the day of operation and some of the drugs should be omitted on the day of operation, so that there are less chances of drug interaction with the drugs used

perioperatively. During preanaesthesia evaluation advice about drug therapy is given.

• There are some conditions, medical or surgical disorders where stress and strain of anaesthesia and surgery is strictly contraindicated for elective and some times emergency operative procedures. In patients with congesive cardiac failure, acute myocardial ischemia or infarction, acute or status asthmaticus, acute liver failure or fulminant hepatitis, acute renal failure, Addison's crisis, Diabetic ketoacidosis or severe dehydration or very critically ill patient, etc, where stabilization of medical disorder is undertaken first an then patient is accepted for operative procedure.

• There are some conditions with life-threatening emergency, one has to accept the patient even though there is high-risk of anaesthesia and surgery like acute trauma or fascio-maxillary injury, head injury, multiple fractures of ribs (flail chest), Tension pneumothorax, obstructed labour, strangulated obstructed hernia, arterial thrombosis, dissceting aneurysms or neonatal emergencies, here one has to accept the patient and accordingly change the convential technique of anaesthesia and perioperative drug therapy.

• To obtain valid written consent for technique of anaesthesia and surgery. Some times there may be problem in taking consent during mass casualties, road traffic accidents, baggers of orfans. Then one should not stick to have valid written consent, one can inform the hospital authority or even consent of two medical personalities present at the time of emergency can be obtained as life saving measure in these patients.

• To ask for preoperative sedation, anxiolytics, control of secretions, control of infection, preoperative blood transfusion whenever necessary, preparation of parts, correction of water and electrolyte imbalance, proper advice is given for all above things for smooth conduction of anaesthesia.

• Again one should give adequate time for evaluating major operative procedures and to patients associated with medical disorders so that preoperative preparation of patient is satisfactory and distribution of time for minor procedures is not wasted. During routine preoperative evaluation and when the operative list is with more number of patients then the distribution of time for all patients (minor and major) should be properly managed so that no patient should be left without assessment and preparation.

All these things can be avoided when these patients are evaluated in the OPD anaesthesia clinic.

Advantages of OPD Anaesthesia clinic

- All the patients either posted for minor or major operative procedures can be evaluated carefully and in details with appropriate advice for investigations as well as for specialist's opinion.
- OPD anaesthesia clinic will provide adequate time for investigations, assessment of reports, opinion of experts of specialists and over all preparation of the patient.
- It will curtail own un-necessary indoor admissions in the hospital.
- With proper guidance in OPD anaesthesia clinic, the patients will get admissions at proper time and unwanted stay in wards will be curtailed down. In turn, it will bring down hospital and Government expenditure and also the expenditure of the relatives of the patient.
- It is of help to reduce the stress and strain of operative procedure in patients and also of relatives by in time admissions and no waiting period in the wards and 11th hour postponement of operation.
- Now a days, to run OPD anaesthesia clinic is important duty of Anaesthesiologist routinely performed, outside the operation theater. At many institutes OPD anaesthesia clinic is running successfully and is of very much help to the patient, surgeons and hospital authorities.

II. INTENSIVE RESIPRATORY CARE UNIT

The Anaesthesiologists play a very important role in the management of patients requiring assisted or artificial mechanical ventilation. This is in view that the anaesthesiologists are well acquainted with respiratory physiology, indications of artificial ventilation, monitoring of patients on artificial ventilation and weaning of patients from mechanical ventilators.

Here in Respiratory Intensive Care unit Anaesthesiologists are concerned with following aspects :

- Construction, staffing and management of Respiratory care unit.
- Assessment of Respiratory parameters, admission in the IRCU, decision whether to keep the patient for only observation, to assist the respiration or control the respiration of patient with appropriate mechanical ventilator, observation and monitoring of patients in IRCU and on ventilators, weaning of patients from artificial ventilation, post-intensive observation in wards and lastly discharge from hospital.
- The anaesthesiologists are concerned with selection of patients to be admitted in respiratory care unit. Here evaluation of the patient for adequacy of respiration, type of respiratory failure, technique of respiratory assistance to be adopted (as whether only to observe, assist or completely control the respiration with mechanical ventilators) and weaning of patient from respiratory therapy.
- Continuous or 24 hours observation and monitoring of the patient on respiratory therapy for proper and timely intervention of technique and in time weaning of patient.
- Anaesthesiologists are well acquanted with mechanical ventilation with the modes of ventilators, the performance and proper selection of ventilators according to indications in that patient and in time weaning form ventilators.

The management of patients in Intensive Respiratory care unit is usually indicated in following circumstances :

1. **Central nervous system**
   - Head injury : Intra-cerebral haemorrhage, subdural or epidural haematoma
   - Cerebro-vascular accidents
   - Unconsciousness or semi-consciousness due to any cause
   - Space occupying lesions
   - Raised intra-cranial tension due to any cause
   - Infections : Meningitis, Encephalitis, cerebral malaria
   - Toxic effects or overdoses of sedatives, narcotic analgesics, intravenous anaesthetic agents, inhalational anaesthetic agents, tranquillizers, cerebral hypoxia, Co_2 narcosis, etc.
   - Poliomyelitis. Ascending polyneuritis, Gullian Barry syndrome

2. **Cardiovascular system**
   - After cardiac arrest due to any cause
   - Congestive cardiac failure
   - Acute myocardial infarction
   - Peripheral circulatory failure due to any cause

3. **Respiratory System**
   - Central or Peripheral respiratory failure
   - Over doses of Sedatives, Narcotic analgesics, drug toxicity on respiratory center
   - Flail chest or chest trauma, multiple fractures of ribs, haemothorax, pneumothorax or tension pneumothorax
   - Status asthmaticus
   - Neuro-paralytic Snake bite
   - Over doses or adverse effects of muscle relaxants
   - Space occupying lesions in mediastinum as hiatus hernia, pleural effusion,
   - Terminal stages of acute hepatic or renal failure
   - Acute Addison's crisis
   - Terminal stages of life

Mechanical or assisted respiratory support is provided by anaesthesiologist and when acute phase is over then weaning of patients from respiratory therapy is done.

III) INTENSIVE CARE UNIT

As the anaesthesiologists are well acquainted to handle emergency situations where resuscitation of the patient is concerned, In Intensive care unit, the patients are very critical and here urgent intervention by expert is necessary to save the life of patient or to decrease the chances of morbidity and mortality as in :

- Quick intravenous access in patients with circulatory collapse or severe trauma and blood loss with un-recordable blood pressure or shock
- Quick endotracheal intubation in patients with respiratory arrest due to any cause, laryngospasm or upper airway obstruction.
- Cardiac thump or external cardiac massage of intra-cardiac injection of Adrenaline in patients with sudden cardiac arrest due to any cause
- Quick and timely intervention to resuscitative steps

Hence anaesthesiologists are specially called in Intensive care unit :

- Intensive Cardiac care unit (ICCU)
- Intensive Respiratory Care Unit (IRCU)
- Intensive Paediatric Care Unit (IPCU)
- Intensive Renal Care Unit
- Intensive Hepatic care unit
- Neonatal Intensive care unit
- Trauma care unit

Now a days Anaesthesiologists are leading the Intensive care area and running the ICUs in private sector.

IV) CARDIO-RESPIRATORY RESUSCITATION

In the operation theater, anaesthesiologists are concerned with handling of emergency situations and institution of quick life support. The eternal vigilance, quick detection, prompt diagnosis and timely treatment, is the part of routine act of anaesthesiologists in the operation theater and monitoring of patient. This specialist's type working pattern of anaesthesiologists is taken as special calling persons to handle emergency situations.

This type of specialized performance skill of anaesthesiologist is many times useful to save the life of patient as well as to reduce the chances of morbidity and mortality peri-operatively or even in wards and casualty. Hence there are very rare chances of perioperative morbidity and mortality in operation theater and in immediate postoperative recovery room.

The anaesthesiologists are specifically called for conduction of cardio-pulmonary resuscitation as they expert in this field. They are supposed to be well concerned with cardio-pulmonary resuscitation (CPR) conduction.

CPR can be under taken as :

    1. Basic life support

    2. Advanced life support

Definition : Cardiac arrest is sudden failure of cardiac action and due to either asystole or ventricular fibrillation.

In general causes of cardiac arrest include :

- Ischemic heart disease
- Drowning
- Electrocution
- Suffocation
- Drug intoxication
- Automobile accidents

1. Basic Life support

It is the emergency first aid procedure that consists of the recognition of airway obstruction, respiratory arrest, cardiac arrest and proper application of cardio-pulmonary resuscitation.

CPR consists of :
- Opening and maintaining patient's airway
- Providing artificial ventilation by means of rescue breathing
- Providing artificial circulation by means of external cardiac compression

2. Advanced life support

It is basic life support with use of adjunctive equipments, intravenous fluid lifeline (infusion) for drug administration, defibrillation, stabilization of victim by cardiac monitoring, control of Dysarrhythmias and post-resuscitation care.

Indications of Resuscitation are :
a) Respiratory arrest
b) *Cardiac arrest* :
   Cardiovascular collapse (electro-mechanical dissociation)
   Ventricular fibrillation
   Ventricular standstill or asystole

Basic life support is an emergency first aid procedure. A maximum sense of urgency is required. It includes A – B – C steps of cardio-pulmonary resuscitation.

Opening of airway and restoring breathing are basic steps of artificial ventilation. The steps can be performed quickly under almost any circumstances and without adjunctive equipments or help of another person.

Establishment of Airway

The initial and most important procedure of successful resuscitation is immediate opening of airway.

Artificial Ventilation

a) Mouth to mouth ventilation
b) Mouth to nose ventilation – when it is difficult to open the mouth and impossible to ventilate via mouth due to facial injury then one must try mouth to nose ventilation.

c) Direct mouth to stoma

d) Self inflating bag and mask or machine

After temporarily starting or assisting ventilation, when patient can not continue his breathing efforts then patient is kept on mechanical ventilators.

Artificial Circulation

- External cardiac compression
- Precordial thump
- Internal cardiac compression
- Defibrillation or cardio version

When sudden , unexpected cardiac arrest occurs, all of A – B – C of basic life support are required in rapid succession. This includes both artificial circulation and artificial ventilation.

Effectiveness of CPR

The reaction of pupils should be checked periodically during CPR, as this provides best indication of Oxygenation. Reaction of pupils indicate adequate oxygenation and blood flow to brain. The carotid pulse should be palpated periodically during CPR so that effectiveness can be assessed.

Precordial Thump

Precordial thump is used in witnessed cardiac arrest (basic life support) monitored patient (advanced life support), pacing and known atrio-ventricular block (advanced life support).

Precautions in Performance of CPR

- Do not interrupt CPR for more than 5 seconds except if endotracheal intubation is already performed.
- Do not move the patient until stabilization and ready for transportation so that un-interrupted CPR during movement is provided.

- Do not compress the xiphoid process at the tip of sternum as laceration of liver can occur.
- In between compressions, release the pressure of hand.
- Body of rescuer should not press the ribs.
- Compression should be smooth, regular and uninterrupted.
- Do not maintain continuous pressure on abdomen.
- The shoulders of rescuer should be directly over the victim's sternum. The elbows should be straight and pressure is applied vertically downwards on lower sternum.
- Usual CPR may result in complications as fracture of ribs, fracture of sternum, costo-chondral separation, Pneumothorax, haemothorax, lung contusion, laceration of liver and fat embolism.
- Special situations are – Drowning, Electric shock and chocking syndrome.

Internal Cardiac compression

When chest is already open, then heart (ventricles) is grasped in between thumb rested at the base of heart inferiorly and index and middle finger at the opposite side of thumb superiorly, or heart is squeezed in the fist of palm. The ventricles are squeezed as quickly as possible within 1 second. This is performed for about 60 – 80 times per minute. It is effective for circulation.

Advanced Life Support

Advanced Life support consists of :
- Initial Basic life support.
- Use of adjunctive equipments, special technics as endotracheal intubation and open chest internal cardiac compression.
- Recognition of Dysarrhythmias and control
- Defibrillation
- Establishment and maintainance of intravenous infusion lifeline
- Employing definitive therapy as correction of acidosis, maintainance of effective cardiac rhythm and circulation.

- Stabilization of patient's condition.
- Basic life support consists clearance of airway, starting of breathing and circulation. In advanced life support along with basic life support, defibrillation and drug therapy is included.
- CPR is necessary at road traffic accidents, natural disasters (fires, earthquakes, fluds, railway or plane accidents, etc)

NEONATAL RESUSCITATION

Neonatal resuscitation is required during caeserean section for obstructed labour, foetal distress, multiple pregnancy, congenital anamolies, premature babies or some times after routine elective vaginal or instrumental delivery.

Anaesthesiologists play an important role in new born resuscitation as they are well acquainted with cardio-pulmonary resuscitation, endotracheal intubation, endobronchial suction for endotracheal secretions. Here the anaesthesiologist are specifically called as there are chances of difficult intubation.

In recent era, neonatal resuscitation should be carried out by expert and promptly as one hand the new born are very precious (only one or two pregnancies is a common practice) and there are chances of permnant neurological deficit if resuscitation is delayed due neuro-behvioural changes secondary to early foetal hypoxia. Scanlon's neuro-behavioural scoring is now preferred over conventional Apgar scoring in new born after normal delivery or caesarean section.

RELIEF OF PAIN AND PAIN CLINIC

As the anaesthesiologists are well acquainted with the relief of pain of all types, in this aspect they are concerned with pain relief during intra-operative, immediate postoperative, chronic and intractable pain.

Their knowledge about the use of analgesics, narcotic analgesics, non-narcotic synthetic analgesics, local anaesthetic agents, various types of nerve blocks, regional anaesthesia techniques and handling of complications related to these, is useful to perform key role in relief of pain.

Now a days. Sophistication, literacy, availability of all measures have compelled the anaesthesiologists to open new doors of practice outside the operation theater. Now relief of pain has gained more importance than conventional practice of anaesthesia inside operation theater. Hence anaesthesiologists (new comers) are either joining already established Pain Clinic or planning to open new clinic serve the mankind.

Relief of pain is concerned with :
1. Acute pain relief
2. Postoperative pain relief
3. Chronic or intractable pain relief

1. Acute pain relief

It deals with any pain acute in onset usually due to trauma, injury any where on the body, accidents, exposure to unaccustomed circumstances, bacterial or viral infection, sudden pneumothorax, dissecting aneurysms, migraine and so on. This type of pain is of short duration, acute in onset and of severe type disturbing normal activity of the person. It is usually treated as treating the causative element an with conventional analgesics or some times narcotic or non-narcotic analgesics or antibiotics.

Here there is no much role to play to anaesthesiologist but in severe cases of migraine, prolapsed disc, fascitis, tension pneumothorax or thrombo-embolic phenomenon, etc. they may be consulted for relief of pain. At these situations potent narcotic analgesics or some times regional anaesthesia blocks may be useful. In case of potent narcotic analgesics use, anaesthesiologists are used to use these drugs so they are called. Here they can tackle the emergency situation when they do occur.

2. Postoperative Pain relief

Intra-operative pain is usually relieved with the drugs used for general anaesthesia or narcotic/non-narcotic analgesics used in balanced anaesthesia technique and with regional anaesthesia.

There is need pain for relief in immediate and late postoperative period which is need of time. Every one is demanding for painless postoperative course. In the minor operative procedures, postoperative pain relief can be provided with simple analgesics, non-narcotic or rarely narcotic analgesics. In major operative procedures or in some indicated patients, postoperative pain relief can be provided as with :

- Potent narcotic or non-narcotic analgesics
- Regional nerve blocks – brachial plexus block, abdominal field block, cervical plexus block, inter-costal nerve block, etc.
- Single shot epidural block
- Continuous epidural block with epidural catheter in thoracic, lumbar or cervical space
- Epidural injection of narcotic or non-narcotic analgesics as Pentazocine, Fentanyl, Morphine, Ketamine, which will provide analgesia for 48 – 72 hours postoperatively.
- Continuous brachial plexus block with catheter in brachial sheath, continuous abdominal field block with catheter can be tried for pain relief.
- During postoperative pain relief, one should monitor vital parameters as pulse rate, blood pressure, adequacy of respiration, hydration, urine out put, toxicity of drugs and over doses which will be better monitored by anaesthesiologists that to after admission in pain clinic. The anaesthesiologists provide postoperative pain relief in wards as part of routine duty outside the operation theater.

3. Chronic or Intractable Pain Relief

Now a day instead of acute or postoperative pain relief, the anaesthesiologists are opting to provide chronic or intractable pain relief. Since last few decades, the relief of intractable pain is gaining more importance than conventional anaesthesia practice inside operation theater. Various techniques in this aspect are being practiced for relief of intractable pain :

- Hypnosis
- Drug therapy : analgesics, anti-histaminics, sedatives or tranquillizers with analgesics, narcotic analgesics

- Trans-cutaneous electrical nerve stimulation
- Various regional blocks
- Regional blocks with neurolytic agents : alcohol, phenol
- Epidural Opioids
- Cryo-analgesia
- Chordotomy

These various techniques of pain relief adopted for intractable pain relief have their own advantages and disadvantages and applicability. Hence through knowledge of various techniques with its applicability in the particular patient is necessary for practice. For this various training programs are being arranged.

Establishment of pain clinic with all facilities, availability all techniques, emergency arrangements if these do occur and experienced persons are necessary to run a pain clinic. In metro politician cities practice of pain clinic is very popular.

OBSTETRIC ANALGESIA

Now a days, painless labour demanded every where. The knowledge about the pain relief as specialty of anaesthesiologists are asked to provide obstetric analgesia. Here the anaesthesiologists are supposed to know about :

- Physiological changes of pregnancy
- Medical disorders associated with pregnancy with its deleterious effect on maternal health and foetal development.
- Placental transfer of the drugs used during obstetric analgesia as well as during obstetric anaesthesia.
- Stages of labour
- Technique of obstetric analgesia to be adopted according to the physical condition of the mother with its indications and applicability as minimum ill-effects on foetus.
- Monitoring of patients during obstetric analgesia.
- In time changeover technique or proceeding with obstetric anaesthesia.

All these clinical pre-requisites and computability of anaesthesiologist, as they are also providing services in this field also. Usually obstetric analgesia is provided with :

- Pharmacological agents : usual analgesics, narcotic analgesics – Morphine, Pethidine, Fentanyl and other.
- Inhalational anaesthetic agents : Oxygen/Nitrous oxide, Air/ Nitrous oxide, Air/Nitrous oxide/Trilene or rarely Oxygen/ Nitrous oxide/Halothane inhalation.
- Epidural block : Single shot or continuous epidural block with Lignocaine or Bupivacaine or mixture of two, Local anaesthetic agents with narcotics – Morphine, Pentazocine, Fentanyl, Ketamine, Tramadol, etc.
- Caudal epidural block with local anaesthetic agents.
- Regional field blocks

Obstetric analgesia is beneficial in reducing stress and strain of labour, psychological insults related to labour, anaesthetic requirement of obstetric anaesthesia, it is of help to decrease morbidity and mortality related to pre-eclampsia or eclampsia. Now to provide obstetric analgesia has become demanding duty of anaesthesiologist outside operation theater.

MISCELLANEOUS DUTIES

a) Now a days the anaesthesiologist are working on their utility in the new zone of Brain Resuscitation. Here intra-cerebral scavenging action of Barbiturates (Thiopentone sodium) is of help to resuscitate the neurons some how and it is under clinical trials with great success. Anaesthesiologists are concerned with intravenous inducing agents as Thiopentone daily so they are of help to work in this regard and also they concerned with critical care, resuscitation and the internal vigilance specialty have compelled them to be leader in this field.

b) In the mental hospitals or Psychiatry centers anaesthesiologists are called to administer anaesthesia for Electro-convulsive therapy. Again here also Thiopentone is of help to analyze the patient's problems and it is helpful for psychoanalysis in prisoners and Police department.

c) Anaesthesiologists are also providing their services in Dental clinics or anaesthesia in dental chair. They are of much help in paediatric dental problems or fascio-maxillary injury.

d) Again anaesthesiologists are called to give anaesthesia in Radiology department, Radiotherapy, Cobalt unit or for CT scan. Here there is problem of anaesthesia in dark, less access of patient during anaesthesia and also face the difficult environment but this is challenging branch to practice anaesthesia outside the operation theater.

e) Again anaesthesiologists are providing their services for Disaster management as situations like floods, Earthquakes, air crash, railway accidents, etc. Mass casualties are better handled by anaesthesiologists due to their working pattern in resuscitation situations, quick approach to patients and timely intervention of emergency services. So they are called with preference.

Thus anaesthesiologists are providing more duties outside the operation theater than conventional anaesthesia in the operation theater for surgical patients. Now there are more and more fields available to work for anaesthesiologists outside the operation theater and which are of more importance for human beings to have safe and cheerful life. They are not behind the curtain which was said to be social drawback in the doctors opting anaesthesia as their specialty after under graduate medical course. No the anaesthesia specialty has become the first choice of postgraduate carrier due to new fields available for practice of anaesthesia than routine practice of anaesthesia inside the operation theater.